"This book begins with a clear and well-articulated explanation of humanistic sandtray therapy, rooted in person-centered gestalt theory. Ryan Foster builds on this as he describes the five phases of HST, clearly explaining theory and how it works in each phase. The chapter on ableism and disabilities is profound. The case examples are as insightful as they are informative. Ryan's detailed applications to many settings and with various populations are extremely thorough and helpful. So much information in this book could be applied to many sandtray approaches. Ryan does an outstanding job of providing a comprehensive guide to HST."

Linda E. Homeyer, PhD, *Distinguished Professor Emerita, Texas State University*

"*Humanistic Sandtray Therapy* will benefit generations of seasoned practitioners as well as those new to the helping professions. Ryan Foster has artfully provided readers with a deep and most practical understanding of humanistic sandtray therapy and its benefits. What is more, he beautifully integrates the theoretical underpinnings of the method."

Rick Carson, *approved supervisor, AAMFT, author of* Taming Your Gremlin *and* A Master Class in Gremlin Taming

"The title of this book says it all—it really is the definitive guide to the why and how of humanistic sandtray therapy. Ryan Foster provides thoroughly engaging and in-depth descriptions of the rationale for HST, the tools needed by practitioners, the process of therapy, and strategies for processing trays with clients. He also addresses neurobiology and trauma in the context of HST and the application of this brilliant modality with multicultural populations, preadolescents and adolescents, people with disabilities, in groups, with couples and families, and in schools and community settings. With humility and humor, he provides practical examples along with guidelines for using HST with clients and in supervision. If you want to learn how to be a humanistic sandtray therapist, this book is an invaluable resource."

Terry Kottman, PhD, LMHC, RPT-S, *director, League of Extraordinary Adlerian Play Therapists*

T0383657

Humanistic Sandtray Therapy

Humanistic Sandtray Therapy: The Definitive Guide to Philosophy, Therapeutic Conditions, and the Real Relationship provides a comprehensive exploration of the underlying theory, necessary skills, and practical applications behind Humanistic Sandtray Therapy (HST) based on a person-centered gestalt model.

This book takes a deep dive into a philosophically based system of sandtray therapy in which all elements of the HST approach are provided in great detail, from the nuts and bolts of creating a sandtray and structuring the experience based on client culture and counseling setting, to process-oriented issues.

Written with a genuine human touch, invaluable materials such as an HST treatment manual and a weblink to videos of HST sessions with real clients are included to assist academics and researchers in designing HST treatment outcome studies.

Ryan D. Foster, PhD, LPC-S, CHST, is associate professor of counseling and department head at Tarleton State University and director of the Humanistic Sandtray Therapy Institute in Fort Worth, Texas.

Humanistic Sandtray Therapy

The Definitive Guide to Philosophy, Therapeutic Conditions, and the Real Relationship

Ryan D. Foster

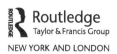

Routledge
Taylor & Francis Group

NEW YORK AND LONDON

Designed cover image: © Getty Images

First published 2025
by Routledge
605 Third Avenue, New York, NY 10158

and by Routledge
4 Park Square, Milton Park, Abingdon, Oxon, OX14 4RN

Routledge is an imprint of the Taylor & Francis Group, an informa business

© 2025 Ryan D. Foster

With contributions from: L. Marinn Pierce, Beck A. Munsey, Ioana Mărcuș, Robin Elkins, James Turnage, Ryan Holliman, and Pedro J. Blanco

The right of Ryan D. Foster to be identified as author of this work has been asserted in accordance with sections 77 and 78 of the Copyright, Designs and Patents Act 1988.

All rights reserved. The purchase of this copyright material confers the right on the purchasing institution to photocopy pages which bear the photocopy icon and copyright line at the bottom of the page. No other parts of this book may be reprinted or reproduced or utilised in any form or by any electronic, mechanical, or other means, now known or hereafter invented, including photocopying and recording, or in any information storage or retrieval system, without permission in writing from the publishers.

Trademark notice: Product or corporate names may be trademarks or registered trademarks, and are used only for identification and explanation without intent to infringe.

ISBN: 9781032660196 (hbk)
ISBN: 9781032658070 (pbk)
ISBN: 9781032664996 (ebk)

DOI: 10.4324/9781032664996

Typeset in Galliard
by Newgen Publishing UK

To Priya, Sahana, and Samuel. Each of you welcomes me into immense here-and-now awareness of how full my heart is with your loving presence and connection.

Contents

Preface

Sandtray therapy is an intervention that was developed when psychoanalysis was the most prevalent form of psychotherapy. It is related to but is not the same as sandplay therapy. Sandtray therapy falls under the broad umbrella of sand therapy and was developed first by Margaret Lowenfield as a way to work with children in much the same way as play therapy. Whereas sandplay therapy is undergirded by Jungian analytical theory, sandtray therapy does not have one unified philosophical base. Therefore, over time, clinicians developed individual ways of using sandtray with clients, often focusing on the power of metaphor and symbolism that the miniatures and the sand held. In the early 2000s, Linda Homeyer and Daniel Sweeney published the first comprehensive guide to sandtray therapy, noting its cross-theoretical application. Their book is now in its fourth edition.

In 2005, I was in my second semester as a master's student in the professional counseling graduate program at Texas State University. I was taking a class called Sandtray Therapy, and I had never heard of sandtray therapy. I was there to satisfy a one-credit-hour requirement for my degree. Linda Homeyer taught the class. She was the first professor I ever had who taught from her own book, the first edition of *Sandtray Therapy: A Practical Manual*. The class was almost totally experiential. We learned the ins and outs of sandtray, and I was hooked. However, I had no opportunity to practice sandtray throughout the rest of my graduate program and into my internship. It remained an interest of mine without a way for me to practically experience it further.

In 2007, I began my doctoral program in counseling at the University of North Texas. Famous for its Center for Play Therapy, its on-campus practicum and internship clinics also had dedicated sandtray rooms. I was excited because I was one of the few students who already had formal training in sandtray. I began using it with adult and adolescent clients for whom I thought sandtray would be appropriate as an adjunct to care, and it worked very well. Still, I did not know how to relate what I was doing in sandtray with my underlying theoretical approach. I felt ungrounded, even though I was practicing what I learned in Linda Homeyer's class.

In 2008, Stephen (Steve) Armstrong published *Sandtray Therapy: A Humanistic Approach*. Steve had an extensive background and training in person-centered and gestalt therapy and, with his book, debuted what is now known as humanistic sandtray therapy (HST). He also happened to be my clinical supervisor at the time, and we clicked on levels both personal and professional. His theoretical sensibilities matched my own, as did his sense of humor and deep care for clients. Yet, I had no idea he was a sandtray therapist who had published his own book. He was humble to the point of self-doubt, often.

Several years later, I landed my first job as a counselor educator at Texas A&M University-Commerce (TAMU-C), where Steve was a faculty member. I began learning of his humanistic model of sandtray therapy and attended trainings at his Sandtray Therapy Institute (STI). Eventually, I became a Certified Humanistic Sandtray Therapist (CHST). Although I moved on professionally from TAMU-C, our relationship transitioned over time from mentor, to mentor and friend, to colleague and friend. He entrusted me with becoming his co-trainer at STI and his only approved CHST supervisor. Eventually, he entrusted me with leading HST trainings and supervising clinicians working toward their CHST. He and I published a series of book chapters and articles on HST, hoping to broaden its audience.

Steve and I had many conversations over the years about HST. At one point, I approached him about my interest in co-authoring a follow-up to his book. He stated that his desire would be to "blow the old book up" and write a replacement book. We talked often about what kind of content we thought would go in the book. I vividly remember meeting with him over Zoom sometime during the COVID-19 pandemic, presenting him with a table of contents I had developed—which is roughly the table of contents in this book—and he liked my outline. However, both of us always seemed to have too much going on to write it.

On June 13, 2022, I texted Steve to say I was using his book, which was self-published and only available for purchase on the STI website, for an expressive arts class I was teaching that summer. I told him that some of my students said they ordered the book a long time ago and had not received it yet. I asked him if there was any way I could help getting them their books from him. I never heard back from him. On June 18, I received a text from his wife, Debbie. She told me that Steve had an accident and was taken to the hospital. I felt worried, but she seemed confident he would be okay. On July 9, I received another text that my mentor, colleague, and dear friend Steve had died from a heart attack. He was six months away from retirement.

I mourned significantly for several months. My grief for the loss of Steve is with me and I access it from time to time; in other moments, I experience what Therese Rando called a subsequent temporary upsurge of grief (STUG). This book is the best way that I can honor Steve and bring to fruition a significant update to the model that he created. It is a project that I struggled to begin because I wanted to make sure that I was thoughtful in my approach to recognizing the incredible mark that his book made on so many people, including me, while also taking a new look at HST.

Therefore, the purpose of this book is to serve as a reconsideration of Steve's original humanistic sandtray model. It is borne out of both of our desires to revisit his model and my desire to create a more explicit description of HST's philosophical assumptions, the characteristic skills, the qualities of the therapeutic relationship, and applications of the model to various populations and therapeutic formats and settings. In addition, I wanted a forum to give other sandtray researchers access to an HST treatment manual I had previously written. Finally, I believe HST fills a wide gap in the field of sandtray because there are not many detailed and theoretically sound sandtray therapies, and I believe after almost 100 years of sandtray therapy's presence, this book might not be a bad idea.

My goal with this book is to support knowledge acquisition and clinical growth of new and experienced sandtray therapists. Although therapists need focused training and experience in order to be an effective sandtray practitioner, I view this text as an essential element in the development of sandtray practice. Therefore, I made a conscious decision to invite co-authors who specialize in using sandtray with diverse populations and in specific clinical settings. Most importantly, I hope clients benefit from sandtray therapists who embody a deep understanding of *why* they do *what* they do in the sand, and my goal is for the information in this book to contribute to that process. From my point of view, healing takes place best in environments and from clinicians who provide ethical, compassionate, and expert care.

Acknowledgements

As I think about all the people who have contributed meaningfully to my growth as a clinician, counselor educator, supervisor, researcher, and author, I feel a rush of deep gratitude. I am going to remark chronologically to the best of my ability, but time has a way of becoming like a plate of mashed potatoes for me. First, I would not have even considered being a psychotherapist if it had not been for two people: Victor Frankl and Nathan Anderson. When I was a high school senior, I was committed to becoming an architect. I had taken several years of construction science and drafting courses, and architecture was the path before me. Nathan, my best friend of now 36 years, and I went to a college open house at a local university. Frankly, we went for the free hotdogs. I met with an architecture advisor and felt overwhelmed with the amount of math involved, and I left feeling disillusioned about the career path I envisioned for myself. Nathan suggested I consider becoming a psychotherapist. I have no idea what he saw in me, but he saw something congruent with the helping professions. Subsequently, I read *Man's Search for Meaning* by Victor Frankl and was completely committed to this idea. These two men changed unequivocally my life path.

When I was a master's student in the professional counseling program at Texas State University, I had numerous mentorship opportunities. Linda Homeyer introduced me to sandtray and play therapy. I really had no idea how important she was to the sandtray therapy field, and after writing this book, I see even more clearly than I ever had before that the world of sandtray therapy would be incredibly different without her. Mike Carns was my professor in a marriage and family therapy survey course as well as an advanced methods course, and he was a master therapist who influenced my clinical judgment and conceptualization. John Garcia called on me out of nowhere in his career counseling course to interpret my Myers-Briggs Type Indicator profile in front of the class—a terrifying notion to me at the time—and subsequently invited me into his world of Jungian thought, where complex thinking became a comfortable place for me. The two people at Texas State who influenced me most to turn toward counselor education and research were Shawn Patrick and John Beckenbach. They allowed me to assist them with research and teaching. John shared a hotel room with me at my first American Counseling Association conference in Detroit and filled my young brain with valuable anecdotes about teaching and research on the plane ride there, during a long walk and cigar break along the streets of Detroit, and during my first poster presentation. These memories are seared into my soul.

As a doctoral counseling student at the University of North Texas (UNT), two professors influenced significantly my clinical, scholarship, and research practice. Jan Holden, who gave me an opportunity to work as her graduate assistant before I even enrolled in my first classes, invited me to first author a chapter in a book she was editing during my first year as a doctoral student. She helped me to feel confident in myself at a time when my self-concept was imminently ready to collapse. My first research agenda was surveying the impact of near-death experiences on bereaved clients, and her mentorship launched me into flight. My dissertation with Jan as my chair was excruciating, and I am a much better writer and thinker because of her. Jan is one of my dearest colleagues and a true friend. Dee Ray gave me another early chance. My second semester, I asked her how a doctoral student gets one of the coveted assistant director positions at the Child and Family Resource Clinic that she directed. She was explicit with the steps and immediately offered me the position, two years away, if I followed those steps. My exposure to clinic administration, assessment, and research molded me into a well-rounded clinician and led me to professional opportunities because of my role at the Clinic. She maintains a supportive and challenging presence in my life and has been there with me every step of the way as I drafted this manuscript.

Many years into my professional life as a counselor educator and clinician, I developed a deep desire to hone my gestalt practice. Steve was part of a gestalt consultation group for many years with Rick Carson, author of *Taming Your Gremlin*, who is a master therapist and gestalt practitioner and supervisor. I had read Rick's book many times based on Steve's suggestion and decided to reach out to Rick on a whim. Fortunately, Rick agreed to provide me with individual training in his Gremlin-Taming Method, and I became a far better therapist and person because of it. It was an intensive ten sessions over many months. Rick's warmth, care, and skill moved me in a way that I have trouble putting into words (perhaps I could place it in a sandtray scene!), and his signature is embedded in the HST method. His focused presence remains with me, and each time I reach out to him to check in, he responds in the same natural, genuine way that defines not only his therapeutic method but also who he is underneath the boundary of his skin.

I co-wrote some of the chapters in this book with practiced sandtray therapists who I have bumped into along the way in my professional life. Ryan Holliman and PJ Blanco are lifelong colleagues and friends whom I first met at UNT. They have served as close peer mentors for almost 20 years, and my experience with them is consistently rich. Beck Munsey is my colleague at Tarleton State University and friend. We have a fantastically genuine relationship in which congruence is a pillar. Ioana Mărcuș and I developed a bond held together by our mutual internal chaos, gestalt theoretical position, and duct tape when we were both assistant professors at Marymount University. Marinn Pierce and I worked closely together while we were board members and presidents of the Association for Spiritual, Ethical, and Religious Values in Counseling, and found common ground in our love for sensory-emotional experiences and seagulls. James Turnage and I immediately connected the first time I met him during a site visit for a mutual graduate student intern supervisee; I saw the sand tray in his office and the miniatures on his shelves and that was it for us. Robin Elkins was my student, licensure supervisee, and humanistic sandtray therapy supervisee. He came prepackaged with a rare mix of intelligence, wisdom, warmth, patience, compassion, love for learning, and inborn clinical ability, and I am proud to call him my co-author.

At the tail end of my preparation of this manuscript, I asked a very special person in my family's life, Anne Showalter, to proofread it. She has given me so much more than noteworthy feedback on this book—she has helped my family and I to bring to life more than this book and I value the essential goodness in her.

Although Steve Armstrong is no longer physically present on Earth, he is housed permanently in my heart and rather active in the secure attachment part of my neurobiology. This book would not exist without the seminal work that he did by creating HST, and my life certainly would be different intrapsychically and professionally had he not invited me into such a meaningful relationship with him. I feel tearful as I write this paragraph—my tears are complex, representing grief, sadness, gratitude, reflection, and love.

My final acknowledgement is to my wife, Priya, daughter, Sahana, and son, Samuel. My heart grew the moment I met Priya ten years ago and, at times, is too large for my ribcage because of our children and the immense love that characterizes our family. I experience safety and security in my family's presence that carries me through each day. They are the reason I have been able to put so much of myself into this book because their authenticity is infectious.

Contributors

Pedro J. Blanco, PhD, LPC-S, RPT-S, CHST, is associate professor of counseling at Tarleton State University in Fort Worth, TX. He has been a practicing therapist using creative approaches to counseling since 2006 and is a certified humanistic sandtray therapist. He is an active researcher and publishes regularly on school-based counseling interventions and play therapy.

Robin Elkins, MS, LPC, CHST, is a trauma therapist for a local mental health agency in Fort Worth, Texas. He has been a practicing certified humanistic sandtray therapist and professional counselor since 2022. He works primarily with individuals diagnosed with IDD and other developmental disabilities.

Ryan Holliman, PhD, LPC-S, RPT-S, is associate professor of counseling at Tarleton State University in Fort Worth, Texas. He has been a professional counselor that utilizes creative approaches since 2010. He is an active researcher in the area of creative approaches in counseling and publishes regularly on these topics.

Ioana Mărcuş, PhD, LPC, NCC, GEP, is a former associate professor of counseling and has been in private practice since 2008. She is the founder of Equibliss Psychotherapy and HEART Space Fund non-profit. Her clinical practice is focused on gestalt equine psychotherapy and other humanistic approaches, including sandtray therapy, to address trauma and eating disorders. She has completed Level II/Advanced training in humanistic sandtray therapy.

Beck A. Munsey, PhD, LPC-S, is associate professor of counseling at Tarleton State University in Fort Worth, Texas. He has been a practicing professional counselor since 2009 and sandtray therapist since 2021. He has completed Level II/Advanced training humanistic sandtray therapy.

His specialty is working with the LGBTGEQIAP+ community, including gender-affirming care.

L. Marinn Pierce, PhD, RYT-200, SEP, is a somatic practitioner in private practice at Embodied Resilience of the Carolinas.

James Turnage, MA, LPC-S, is clinical director for disability services for a local mental health authority in Tarrant County, Texas. He has experience providing counseling and management services in a children's advocacy center, domestic violence shelters, community crisis center, community mental health centers, and disability programs. He has worked for 18 years serving as program manager for an adult outpatient clinic, director of child/adolescent services, clinical director for adult outpatient clinics, and clinical director for disability division. He has been a practicing sandtray therapist for 20 years.

About the Author

Ryan D. Foster, PhD, LPC-S, CHST, is associate professor of counseling and department head at Tarleton State University in Fort Worth, Texas and has been a counselor educator since 2010. He is also director of the Humanistic Sandtray Therapy Institute in Fort Worth, where he trains mental health practitioners in humanistic sandtray therapy that can lead to the Certified Humanistic Sandtray Therapist (CHST) credential. In addition, he is an active private practice counselor. Dr. Foster has published more than 20 articles and chapters in the fields of sandtray therapy and transpersonal experiences in counseling, as well as an edited book on spiritual practices in counseling. He is the author of the *Humanistic Sandtray Therapy Treatment Manual* and has served on the editorial boards of *Counseling and Values* and the *World Journal for Sand Therapy Practice*.

Visit the Humanistic Sandtray Therapy Institute's website at www.humanisticsandtray.com for a host of useful videos.

Part I

The Humanistic Sandtray Therapy Framework and Process

Chapter 1

Theoretical and Philosophical Tenets of Humanistic Sandtray Therapy

Sand therapy practice has been around for about a century. Its development parallels the growth of traditional talk therapy, and its popularity has increased exponentially in the last 20 years. Sand therapy is generally separated into two categories: sandplay therapy and sandtray therapy (Homeyer & Lyles, 2022). *Sandplay therapy* refers specifically to a Jungian approach to sand therapy and is based on Dora Kalff's (1971) standardization and theoretical formulation of Margaret Lowenfeld's (1950, 2007) World Technique. Sandtray therapy is a broad term that encompasses a variety of philosophical approaches to working with clients using a tray of sand and miniature figures (Homeyer & Lyles, 2022; Homeyer & Sweeney, 2023). For a detailed history of the development of sand therapies and their assorted terminology, I refer you to Chapter 1 in Homeyer and Lyles (2022).

All sand therapies share elements that seem universal in terms of how they contribute therapeutically. Sand therapies, in their most basic forms, assist clients in telling their stories within a safe psychotherapeutic environment (Homeyer & Lyles, 2022; Homeyer & Sweeney, 2023). In addition, the use of metaphor in a three-dimensional world is unique to sand therapies, and, unlike traditional talk therapy, sand therapies are unreliant on verbal communication singularly. Also, sand therapies can be used across developmental spectrums with an incredibly wide variety of diverse populations. However, there are notable differences between sandplay and sandtray therapy, particularly in terms of philosophy. In my experience, for the therapist who is new to sand therapy, it can be rather confusing to delineate what sets sandtray therapy apart from sandplay—often because, historically, authors and practitioners have used the terms interchangeably. Bradway (1996, 2002, 2006) strongly encouraged sand therapy practitioners to attend to nuance and stop synonymizing sandplay and sandtray. Others have made attempts at providing clear definitions for sand therapy, sandplay, and sandtray (Dawson, 2024; Homeyer & Lyles, 2022; Homeyer & Sweeney, 2023); unfortunately, based on my review of the extant literature,

DOI: 10.4324/9781032664996-2

practitioners and authors have yet to follow suit fully with these expert suggestions.

Unlike sandplay therapy, sandtray therapy is not based on a singular theoretical orientation and is a non-standardized approach. Even newer approaches that claim to have strength in having an underlying theoretical rationale, such as Fleet's (2023) pluralistic sandtray therapy, seem to focus far more on how to work with clients or what sandtray may be activating psychologically in clients than conceptual logic of sandtray procedures and processes. In contrast, Homeyer and Sweeney (2023) developed one of the most cited and highly regarded models of sandtray therapy and described it as cross-theoretical, meaning that therapists "can integrate a wide variety of theoretical and technical psychotherapeutic approaches" (p. 1). In addition, they emphatically stated that "the use of sandtray therapy should always be theoretically based … techniques without theory are reckless, and [have the] potential to be damaging" (p. 1). Theory is like a guidebook (Fall, Holden, & Marquis, 2023) and its place is to help therapists make sense of their clients, the therapeutic process, clinical decisions, and technical applications.

Homeyer and Lyles (2022) noted three non-Jungian theoretically sound approaches from their review of literature—Narrative Sand Therapy© (Preston-Dillon, 2009), Adlerian sandtray play therapy (Kottman, 2023), and the model on which this book expands, humanistic sandtray therapy (Armstrong, 2008). In addition, Day and Day (2012) described a model of sandtray therapy based on transactional analysis. Dawson (2024) provided a model of sandtray therapy grounded in internal family systems and polyvagal theory. In practice, most therapists who employ sandtray therapy tend to come from humanistic or Adlerian backgrounds (Boik & Goodwin, 2000). Moreover, Homeyer and Lyles (2022) predicted that, "as the future unfolds, there will be more theoretically-sound approaches and applications to sandtray therapy. The field needs innovation and growth" (p. 12). Likely, the field of sandtray therapy will continue to mature as more practitioners seek training and supervision in one or more sandtray approaches.

Humanistic sandtray therapy (HST; Armstrong, 2008) developed out of a need for humanistically oriented therapists to launch their sandtray practice from a familiar and secure philosophical base. It is a complete system of sandtray therapy that can be used either as an adjunct to therapeutic care or as the primary method by which client healing takes place. Of note is that many elements of Homeyer and Sweeney's (2023) cross-theoretical model of sandtray synchronize seamlessly with HST, and those interested in HST should also review their text. Before focusing on *how* a therapist operates in HST, it is important to understand the *why* underlying the elements of this approach. Without a sound, consistent way of perceiving, not only the application of sandtray, but also the client's inner world of experiencing, context, background, and the role of the therapeutic relationship, the therapist will be traveling alongside the client without basic tools of navigation. In their classic examination of psychotherapy mechanics, Frank and Frank (1991) described a set of components shared by all approaches:

1. A confidential and "emotionally charged" (p. 40) relationship with a helper
2. This relationship is in a healing environment
3. There is systematic and theoretical logic that explains the client's symptoms and provides a method of healing that both the client and the helper must accept
4. This method requires active engagement of the client and helper, is based on the systematic logic, and requires buy-in from both client and helper.

HST is more than a technique or method; it is a model in which all elements are based on theoretical rationale and aligns with the characteristics noted by Frank and Frank.

Humanistic sandtray therapy is defined as *a dynamic, experiential philosophical approach to sandtray therapy grounded in a synthesis of person-centered and gestalt theories in which the power of the here and now is harnessed to invite clients into increased awareness and paradoxical change.* Practitioners of the HST approach can be described best as person-centered gestaltists (Herlihy, 1985). Person-centered and gestalt theories, although different in technical implementation, share several philosophical tenets:

1. A Maslovian foundation based on the self-actualizing tendency
2. The value of discovery learning
3. The essence of the therapeutic process as experiencing
4. Emphasis on the creation of an authentic and trusting I/Thou relationship
5. Attention to the genuineness of the therapist as a person
6. The need for therapists to be with clients while retaining their own separateness
7. The belief that their approaches, widely applied, would benefit both the individual and society (Herlihy, 1985, p. 21).

All humanistic approaches to psychotherapy value growth, acceptance, empathy, authenticity, presence, and congruence. In addition, humanistic psychotherapists center their efforts on development and maintenance of the therapeutic relationship above all other factors in psychotherapy;

decades of research support the notion that the therapeutic relationship is the single most significant agent of change on which therapists have the most influence (Wampold & Imel, 2015). However, in addition to the influence of the therapeutic relationship, humanistic sandtray therapists believe that the HST process can be a meaningful invitation for a client's growth and change. My goal in this text is to elucidate fully the why, what, and how of HST so that mental health practitioners, researchers, educators, and students have access to a complete system of sandtray therapy. To begin, in this chapter, I will discuss traits that contribute to the power of sandtray work in a humanistic context. Then, I will outline philosophical and theoretical underpinnings of HST in terms of human nature, maladaptive functioning, and healing. Finally, I will share essential qualities of humanistic sandtray therapists.

The Power of Humanistic Sandtray Therapy

Sandtray is the medium (Allan & Berry, 1987) that is used for clients to express their phenomenological worlds. HST is the holistic process that transacts before, during, and after use of sandtray. HST shares several general process traits with other forms of sandtray therapy (Homeyer & Sweeney, 2023), and my intention here is to discuss these overlapping concepts from a humanistic point of view. HST can be categorized as an expressive therapy (ET; Pearson & Wilson, 2009) and, therefore, aligns well with five traits that make ET so powerful therapeutically: HST is sensory, indirect, inclusive, cathartic, metaphoric, and it promotes therapeutic depth (Armstong, 2008; Armstrong et al., 2017).

Sensory Experience in HST

HST provides clients with opportunities to get their body involved, activating kinesthetic sensory awareness (Armstrong, 2008). Perhaps even more importantly, it allows them to connect to, experience, and perceive motion and where their bodies are in space. Armstrong et al. (2017) noted that "[s]andtray is sensual and many clients of all ages touch the sand throughout the sandtray therapy session" (p. 228). Homeyer and Sweeney (2023) stated that "[t]he very tactile experience of touching and manipulating the sand is a therapeutic experience in and of itself" (p. 15). Interacting with sand can bring up both positive and negative experiences and memories, grist for the therapeutic mill, in a way that traditional talk therapy simply cannot. In addition, clients can experience the physical nature of the sandtray miniatures. and acts of touching and arranging these objects in their trays may evoke clients' emotions. I have witnessed clients and supervisees spend a considerable amount of time getting their sandtray scenes just the way they want them to ensure their perceptions are accurately represented, connecting their minds and bodies. For clients who have visual impairment or other sensory limitations, involving their bodies can be especially important.

Indirect Expression in and Inclusivity of HST

When I train clinicians and graduate students in HST, I often tell them that HST can be a side door into a client's world. Although all clients come into therapy with defenses intact to an extent, humanistic sandtray can bypass some obstacles to fully understanding and empathically attuning with a client's experiences. Sometimes clients feel safer expressing themselves and telling their stories of pain, loss, trauma, and conflict through their sandtray scenes (Armstrong, 2008). Going to therapy can be terrifying, especially when clients bring in assumptions that if they talk about their hurt, they may never be able to escape it. For other clients, the non-verbal nature of sandtray creation and observation may align well with their developmental level (Homeyer & Sweeney, 2023) or for clients who have a communication limitation based on an ability difference (Smith, 2012; see Chapter 8 for more on this topic). Other clients are unable to find the words for their experiences and depicting them in metaphor can appropriately capture the depths of their backgrounds, perceptions, and feelings.

Cathartic Experience in HST

Armstrong (2008) defined catharsis in HST as "an intense expression of emotion previously unexpressed and sometimes previously outside of awareness" (p. 11). HST may provoke clients to experience deep emotion and catch them by surprise because of the indirect nature of this approach. I have had many experiences with clients who are tearful upon creating their scenes without having spoken a word about their trays. Other times, I have witnessed catharsis when clients shift their focus to a certain miniature in or area of their scenes. Catharsis may involve sadness, fear, conflict, anger, joy, disgust, or a sense of ambivalence or confusion.

Metaphor

Sandtray scenes and their related elements are metaphorical by nature. Metaphor is used in many therapeutic approaches and sometimes is provided by the therapist. I use metaphor often in talk therapy sessions; sometimes therapist-provided metaphors land and sometimes they do not. In HST, however, "clients create their *own* metaphors in the sand, [so] therapists have a symbol that is formed *by clients*. Therefore, therapists do not have to worry if clients will relate to the metaphor" (Armstrong, 2008, pp. 11–12; italics his). Metaphor allows clients to capture their experiences in ways that can make the therapeutic process more efficient. One sandtray scene may provide more contextual information, including cultural background (Homeyer & Sweeney, 2023), than could be gathered in a single session of talk therapy. Additionally, metaphor allows clients to observe themselves from a different angle, thus increasing their awareness and self-understanding; this is especially powerful when therapist and client stay with and work in the metaphor of the tray (see Chapter 4 for further discussion of this topic). Metaphor also allows for access to themes to emerge, much like in child-centered play therapy (Landreth, 2023).

Promotion of Therapeutic Depth in HST

Armstrong (2008) stated that HST "fosters deeper self-disclosure" (p. 12). Because HST provides a holistic sensory experience, is indirect and inclusive, provokes catharsis, and is metaphorical by nature, clients are exposed to new depths of their experiences. As I will discuss later in this chapter, because the HST focus is on here-and-now awareness, exploration, and discovery, humanistic sandtray therapists are not trying to take the client further than they are in the moment. HST invites clients to enter a space of *simply noticing* (Carson, 2003) in potentially unfamiliar ways. This approach exposes clients to their own immediate experiencing in ways that can lead them to discovering hidden emotions, bodily awareness, self-perception, and unfinished business. Due to the potential for significant therapeutic intensity during HST, humanistic sandtray therapists can empathically attune deeply to clients' experiences, thereby contributing to the quality of the therapeutic relationship as well as a growth-orientation. I discuss how humanistic sandtray therapists conceptualize these important aspects of clients next.

Human Nature

To successfully apply HST, it is critical to understand with what capacities humans are born into the world. Having a grasp of human nature assists humanistic sandtray therapists with maintaining a sense of optimism and hope, a critical attitude in the therapeutic environment (Yalom, 1980), because of a strong emphasis on the growth-orientation of human beings. Understanding these concepts also assists humanistic sandtray therapists with grasping clients' internal worlds. One of the "pillars of gestalt" (Yontef, 1999, p. 11) is phenomenology, defined as "[t]he search for understanding through what is obvious and/or revealed, rather than through what is interpreted by the observer" (Mann, 2021, p. 8). Thus, of primary interest to humanistic sandtray therapists is clients' inner experiencing—*what is obvious*—rather than the therapist's *interpretation* of clients' worlds. This pillar applies to process and content inside and outside of the tray. Approaching sandtray therapy from a humanistic base of philosophical assumptions allows sandtray therapists to conceptualize clients' processes in the context of their situation or environment. In this section, I review core concepts of human nature that are fundamental to HST, including the actualizing tendency, contextual freedom of choice, the capacity for immediate experiencing, and field theory. Before moving forward, however, I provide a caveat: The following discussion serves as a summary of principles and concepts arising from person-centered and gestalt theories. For a complete understanding, I encourage you to take a deeper dive into the references provided at the end of the chapter.

The Actualizing and Self-actualizing Tendency

Humanistic sandtray therapists believe that all humans are born with an innate capacity for growth, known as the actualizing tendency (Rogers, 1957). Rogers (1951) stated that people have "one basic tendency and striving—to actualize, maintain, and enhance the experiencing organism" (p. 487). It is a holistic internal mechanism that propels people forward toward survival, growth, autonomy, relationships with others, and functional behaviors (Wilkins, 2016). Relatedly, the self-actualizing tendency (Rogers, 1959) is an inborn process that reflects the extent to which people experience themselves as responding to the actualizing tendency. Parallel to Rogers, Perls (1959) also acknowledged humans' inborn capacity for actualization, stating that "every individual … has only one inborn goal—to actualize itself as it is" (p. 33). In HST, therapists emphasize leaning into and activating clients' actualizing tendency by partnering with them in their growth.

Holism

Holism is another core philosophical assumption of HST. Its meaning is best captured in the relative translation of gestalt, which is "pattern, form, shape, whole configuration" (Mann, 2021, p. 7). Psychologically and perceptually, people are composed of meaningful wholes. People are who they are because of a total pattern. Gestalt psychology compels humanistic sandtray therapists to reject the notion that people can be treated as though they are made of various identifiers on a demographic form. It is true that a person's background history, early childhood experiences, traumas, culture, and current issues or needs are important to understanding a person as well as a person's understanding of self, for example. However, humanistic sandtray therapists view each person as a patterned whole who has been influenced by each of these factors. Fall et al. (2023) used the metaphor of a chocolate chip cookie to explain the concept of gestalt. When one eats a chocolate chip cookie, one tastes what is known as a chocolate chip cookie. Its taste is fundamentally different from that of a sugar cookie, even though the basic ingredients of both cookies are the same: butter, flour, eggs, sugar, and baking soda. One does not taste the individual ingredients in either of the cookies. In addition, no two chocolate chip cookies, even out of the same batch, will taste the same because of the individual cookie's ingredient load (e.g.., the amount of any one ingredient that was captured in each cookie) and position on the cookie sheet while in the oven. One tastes the whole (delicious) unique cookie! Therefore, humanistic sandtray therapists view each client as a total, whole person, leading them to treat every client as they are now, as therapists interact with them, moment to moment. Just as a cookie changes as the minutes, days, and hours pass, so people do. Therefore, humanistic sandtray therapists open themselves to perceive their clients as they are in the here and now.

Field Theory

Lewin's (1951) field theory is another pillar of gestalt theory (Mann, 2021; Yontef, 1999), captured in the following formula:

$$B = f(P,E)$$

translated as *behavior (B) is a function of the person (P) and their environment (E)*. People interact simultaneously and dynamically with their internal and phenomenal external environment, also referred to as a situation (Mann, 2021). For example, my little white dog, Joey, barks at every delivery person who drops off a package at my house. It is typical for me to sharply raise my voice and say, "Be quiet!" to Joey. Here, the ways in which I am engaging with my perception of Joey's barking reciprocally are the *situation*. I have lots of options to reach out to my world/Joey and his barking each time it takes place. When it is just Joey and me in the middle of the day, my voice is minimally sharp and at a moderately raised volume. When Joey barks at 8:00 p.m. after my 5-year-old daughter has just fallen asleep, then I express more of a "quiet yell," with tremendous sharpness. My voice tone and sharpness are quite related to my immediately present mood, too!

In HST, field theory allows therapists to view clients' responses as inter-relations between themselves and their phenomenological perception of their situation or environment, which includes their here-and-now relation-ship and interaction with their environment. A client's situation can include other people, relationships, objects, dreams, or their fantasies, to name just a few components. Importantly, a client's situation also includes their sandtray scene. Humanistic sandtray therapists make concerted attempts to understand their clients based on field theory, meaning that therapists cannot separate people from their interactions with their situations, which are dynamic and flowing (Parlett, 1991). Therefore, in HST, there is a dynamic and reciprocal process between clients and their sandtray scenes. Clients' perceptions of their scenes are in flux and may change during a single sandtray session. New awareness may also emerge over time as clients bring up past sandtray scenes to their therapists.

Awareness, Contact, and Contact Boundaries

Awareness and contact are fundamental processes that are inherent to human beings (Perls, Hefferline, & Goodman, 1951/1994). Awareness lies on a continuum (Mann, 2021) and refers to one's sense of being with what is, without judgment, in the here and now, as one engages with a situ-ation. Awareness is interrelated with one's environment. Because awareness lies on a spectrum, and engages with a given situation, one may or may not be completely in contact with one's whole experience in the moment. For example, when I am loading my washing machine with this week's laundry, I may be in dulled contact with the here and now. However, when I am facilitating a sandtray session with a client, I attempt to remain vibrantly aware in the moment.

Contact refers to people's ongoing meaning-making processes as they reach out toward their environment while the environment impacts them (Perls et al., 1951/1994). Contact involves the five senses, our physiology, and our perceptions and judgment. People are always in contact and main-tain a relationship with their environment. How people react and respond to the messages and meanings they receive from their environment is based on how they shift their awareness. Contact may happen with people, nature, sounds, memories, dreams, animals, hopes, and disappointments, to name some examples. Contact is not togetherness, but it is interactional (Polster & Polster, 1973). Good contact—that is, a flexible and open sense of awareness and receptivity to the environment while maintaining a sense of separation—can lead to creativity, new discoveries, relational attunement to others, self- and other understanding, and even insight. Humanistic sandtray therapists provide a space in which good contact can happen with their clients, sandtrays, and the psychotherapy situation.

Relatedly, the contact boundary is the threshold of differentiation at a person's sense of self and the environment. Polster and Polster (1973) defined the contact boundary as "the point at which one experiences the 'me' in relation to that which is not 'me' and through this contact, both are more clearly experienced" (pp. 102–103). As people make attempts to self-regulate, they experience the environment as supportive, toxic, or somewhere in between and change contact boundary permeability to modify the degree of influence the environment has on self: impermeable in response to perceptually toxic environments, and permeable in response to perceptually supportive environments.

In person-centered and gestalt theory, people's needs are organismic (Pearls, Hefferline, & Goodman, 1951/1994; Rogers, 1942), reflecting "the lived quality of experience" (Mann, 2021, p. 10). People inherently aim toward *organismic self-regulation* as needs arise that may call for immediate satisfaction or require longer-term completion. The nature of needs can be understood through the figure and ground relationship and the awareness-excitement-contact cycle (Zinker, 1977).

Figure, Ground, and the Awareness-Excitement-Contact Cycle

Figure is "what surfaces for [a person] at any given moment" (Mann, 2021, p. 15). When I eat a chocolate chip cookie, my figure is the scent of the cookie, the way it feels in my mouth as I chew it, and its chocolatey goodness. Ground is a person's "entire experience of the world from [their] early upbringing, … embodied cultural beliefs, … education, … what [they] had for lunch—[their] entire experience of [their] world to date including [their] imaginings for the future" (p. 15).

As I eat my chocolate chip cookie, my ground is composed of my experiences of my wife's homemade cookies and what her baking symbolizes to me—an act of care and love—as well as how many cookies I imagine I will eat to satisfy my hunger for a snack. My ground is also made of my past struggles with sugar intake and overall nutritional health; therefore, I may feel anxious as I think about eating another cookie. Like other concepts in humanistic theory, figure and ground are in flux. A person's ground influences emergence of new figures and vice versa. Figure and ground are reciprocal. However, only one figure may be present in a person's awareness at any one moment in time.

The awareness-excitement-contact cycle (Zinker, 1977) is a model of the gestalt cycle of experience that provides humanistic sandtray therapists with a map illuminating how figures emerge out of ground and needs come to completion. Gestalt cycles may be brief or may happen over a period of years or decades and are psychophysiological in nature. People also have cycles within cycles (Mann, 2021). The first point in this cycle is *sensation*, during which a person becomes aware of a need, typically arising physiologically. *Awareness* then arises, allowing the person to understand what their need is and how to accomplish it. Next, the person enters *mobilization*, in which they ready themselves, often creating the psychophysiological energy warranted to satisfy their need. Once mobilized, the person carries out the *action* required of their body and mind. They arrive then at *contact*, which is the active process of engaging with the environment. The final point in the cycle is *satisfaction*, in which the need cycle is completed, and the person enters a stage of "withdrawal, of relaxation, recuperation, disinterest" (Zinker, 1977, p. 92). Thus, homeostatic balance (Perls et al., 1951/1994) is attained. A new figure emerges, and the cycle begins again.

To demonstrate the cycle, I will provide an example. As I am writing the above paragraph, I experience a *sensation* of restlessness in my chest and my legs. I become *aware* that I have a need to get out of my chair and take a walk. I mobilize myself by completing the paragraph, think about where I want to walk—on my treadmill or in my neighborhood—and decide to walk outside. I take *action* by lifting myself out of my chair, walk out of the door, lock the door, and walk toward the street in front of my house. I *contact* my environment by taking my usual 10-minute walk around the block, taking one step at a time at a brisk pace. I then arrive back home and enter my front door, finding that my need to walk is *satisfied*. I engulf myself in a feeling of disinterest in any further exercise. Now, I begin to sense a dry mouth and sweat running down the back of my neck, and I have arrived at the first point in a new cycle.

Freedom and Responsibility

Humanistic sandtray therapists believe that people have contextual freedom of choice due to their innate actualizing tendency, organismic self-regulation process, and capacity for awareness. People are free to become actively engaged in their own sense of awareness and, therefore, more fully develop their potential. Moreover, Cain (2002) stated that "[h]umanistic therapists view people as essentially free to choose the manner and course of their living and their attitude toward events. At the same time that people are free to choose, they are also responsible for their choices" (p. 12). People are faced with choices in each moment and with each breath (Carson, 2003). Because people cannot be removed from their environment, however, people's choices can be limited by their relationship with their environments. Assuredly, there are fundamental differences among and between people in the level of toxicity of the environment, and these differences will have a major impact on choice. For example, because I am a White, middle-class, heterosexual, cisgender male who is able-bodied, I experience access to a wider array of choices because I am in contact with a generally supportive societal environment due to my privileged identities.

Maladaptive Functioning

Although people are born into the world with an actualizing tendency that moves them toward lifelong growth and the potential for organismic self-regulation, they do not exist in a vacuum. People and their environments are constantly in meaningful and imperfect relation. Everyone faces internal and external challenges at different points in their lives. Of interest here is what leads to maladaptive functioning, reactions, and responses according to humanistic philosophy. In this section, I discuss contact boundary disturbance, incongruence, and unfinished business.

Contact Boundary Disturbances

Fall et al. (2023) stated that "maladjustment occurs when, in the face of an environment chronically unsupportive of need fulfillment, one responds to anxiety by restricting awareness" (p. 230). By nature, contact boundaries lie on a continuum of permeability as people try to sift through experiences in their environment that are either toxic or supportive. In functional contact boundaries, people dynamically connect with environments that are supportive and withdraw from environments that are toxic. When people experience environments that are persistently toxic, they develop patterns of *contact boundary disturbances* in which they disown awareness via their continuum of permeability (Yontef, 1993). On one end of the permeability continuum is complete permeability, called confluence, in which people fuse self with other/situation/environment. On the other end of permeability is complete impermeability, called isolation, in which people lose all contact between self and other/situation/environment.

Yontef (1993) identified four types of contact boundary disturbances. The first is *retroflection*, which is when self is split into warring parts. In retroflection, people do to themselves what they wish to do outside of self, maybe even *to* someone else. Therefore, in their efforts to shut themselves down from their environment, they end up isolating. For example, instead of discussing tension-filled issues with me or others in my family of origin, my dad has established a pattern of leaving the room and silently introspecting alone as a response to his own anger and other vulnerable feelings. In *introjection*, people absorb material from their environment without filtering. They demonstrate great permeability in their boundaries, while developing a rigid personality style. People whose contact boundaries are patterned by introjection respond according to a system of rules and values for which they hold themselves tightly accountable. For example, when I was a young psychotherapist, I would often respond to clients using the exact words that my professors and clinical supervisors said in class or during supervision, without attending to the context or meaning of those responses for my clients.

Projection is common in therapeutic parlance. In projection, people confuse self and other/situation/environment by "attributing to the outside something that is truly self" (Yontef, 1993, p. 138). People who tend to avoid responsibility for their own feelings, thoughts, or behaviors are engaging in projection. For example, it is common at academic institutions for lower-level administrators to blame higher-level administrators for decisions that they believe faculty members will perceive as negative, instead of the lower-level administrators owning their own perceptions of such moves. Finally, *deflection* is "the avoidance of contact or of awareness by turning aside" (Yontef, 1993, p. 138). Toxic positivity, the belief that people should maintain a positive attitude no matter how difficult life gets, is one example of deflection. Clients often symbolize contact boundary disturbances in their sandtray scenes by creatively arranging fences, walls, stones, or gems.

Incongruence and the Zeigarnik Effect

In HST, contact boundary disturbances lead to incongruence. *Incongruence* is the state of "discrepancy between the self as perceived and the actual experience of the organism" (Wilkins, 2016, p. 49). Incongruence is what brings people into therapy and, as I discuss later in this chapter, is a necessary condition for client healing via psychotherapy. It is the underlying force that leads to tension, anxiety, and problematic behaviors. Conceptually, incongruence is strongly influenced by a gestalt concept known as the Zeigarnik effect, commonly known as unfinished business (Mann, 2021). The Zeigarnik effect postulates that people inherently seek completion of their gestalts. They want to make "meaningful wholes for their experience even when that experience was incomplete" (p. 85). According to the Zeigarnik effect, people's lives are filled with instances of unfinished business, which are essentially incomplete gestalts. Unfinished business can be contextually minor, such as when I leave the dishes undone sometimes before I go off to relax for the evening, to major, such as pervasive feelings of loss related to the death of my sister. In HST, unfinished business is often symbolized as one of the main features of clients' sandtray scenes.

Healing

In humanistic sandtray therapy, there are two core principles undergirding the nature of healing in psychotherapy. Almost all therapists are familiar with the first principle: Client growth and change hinge on the quality of the therapeutic relationship between client and therapist. Decades of research also support the notion that the therapeutic relationship is a fundamental agent of client change (Wampold & Imel, 2015). The second core principle in HST is that healing is an experiential process based on paradox. I will explore both principles by examining Rogers' (1957) core conditions, gestalt relational concepts, and the paradoxical theory of change (Beisser, 1970).

The Therapeutic Relationship

A core postulate in HST is that the therapeutic relationship is a necessary condition. *A deep relational connection must exist between therapist and client prior to engaging in humanistic sandtray work* (Armstrong, 2008). With younger clients, sandtray can act to facilitate the establishment of a therapeutic relationship (more on this topic in Chapter 6). Unless an adult or adolescent client makes a specific request to engage in sandtray therapy—and I have experienced this situation to my surprise (and delight!)—I tend to focus on developing the therapeutic relationship, following my typical non-sandtray humanistic therapy protocol. Because the relationship structures the entirety of the psychotherapy process, I will discuss integral assumptions including Rogers' (1957) core conditions, gestalt concepts of contact as it applies to the therapeutic relationship, dialogue, and inclusion.

Conditions of Personality Change

Rogers' (1957) six conditions of personality change lie at the heart of healing in HST. Although Rogers believed that these conditions were necessary *and* sufficient—meaning that when these conditions were satisfied, client change would emerge inherently—in HST, they function as necessary *but not* sufficient for client change. However, these conditions build the foundation of a safe therapeutic relationship and lasting client change cannot take place without them in HST. A therapist can have the most magnificent sandtray miniatures collection in the universe, but without a therapeutic relationship based on Rogers' conditions, there will be no client change. In addition, it seems that many therapists tend to view the core conditions as something that can achieve permanency. On the contrary, the core conditions are an ever-flowing dynamic for which therapist and client share responsibility to create, maintain, re-create, and re-maintain over time and context. Below, I summarize each of the core conditions.

The first condition is that the client and therapist are "in psychological contact" (Rogers, 1957, p. 96). The humanistic sandtray therapist's presence is fundamental to making psychological contact. However, the client must also be open to receiving contact from the therapist. Both therapist and client must create permeability in their contact boundaries for successful psychological contact to take place.

Condition two requires the client to be "in a state of incongruence" (Rogers, 1957, p. 96). This condition may seem obvious to some therapists. However, condition two can be complex because a client may be shielding themselves from their own incongruence. They may put up a front that they are okay and conclude that therapy has little chance of helping them. In addition, some clients arrive to their first session of psychotherapy in an involuntary capacity—children and adolescents are a common example of involuntary clients. On the other hand, some clients arrive ready to do the work of psychotherapy because they have been in a state of misery for as long as they can remember. For HST, I do not recommend attempting to use sandtray with clients who have created resistance to their own incongruence. Fulfillment of this condition precedes not only a good therapeutic relationship, but also good sandtray work.

The third condition necessitates therapist congruence (Rogers, 1957), also referred to as "genuineness or realness" (Armstrong, 2008, p. 21). Rogers (1989) considered congruence as by far the most important condition. Rogers (1957) stated that congruence "means that within the relationship he is freely and deeply himself, with his actual experience accurately represented by his awareness of himself" (p. 97). It is essential for humanistic sandtray therapists to show up with an openness toward their own vulnerability so that they are not hiding themselves from their clients. Genuine therapists show up fully for their clients and present with their own experiences. I highly recommend that therapists find their own good therapist with whom they can do meaningful resolution of unfinished business, increase their own awareness, and nurture their organismic self-regulation and actualizing tendency. In my 15 years of being a clinical supervisor and counselor educator, I have noticed that therapists who have not engaged in personal therapy are limited in their ability to maintain congruence with clients. When therapists are distracted by their own patterns of resistance, a safe therapeutic relationship cannot be established because the therapist is not being real with their clients and, therefore, are unable to co-create a *real relationship*.

The fourth condition requires the therapist's unconditional positive regard (UPR; Rogers, 1957) from the client. Rogers defined UPR as "the extent that the therapist finds himself experiencing a warm acceptance of each aspect of the client's experience as being a part of that client" (p. 98). In HST, therapists avoid projecting expectations, conditions, or "shoulds" onto their clients, and instead openly accept the client for not only who they are, but also how they experience themselves.

Condition five captures the therapist's experience and communication of empathy to the client (Rogers, 1957) in which empathy is defined as such: "To sense the client's private world as if it were your own, but without ever losing the 'as if' quality" (p. 99). It is not enough for the therapist to experience empathy, however. They must also attempt to "both communicate his understanding of what is clearly known to the client and can also voice meanings in the client's experience of which the client is scarcely aware" (p. 99). In my experience, when I am more open, vulnerable, and real with a client, I can receive them with clarity and experience deep empathy. However, sometimes it is not so easy to communicate empathy to a client, because it requires nuanced meanings and emotions. The client's sandtray scene can be a great help in providing clarity to the therapist searching to communicate empathy to a client.

Condition six necessitates that "the client perceives, to a minimal degree, the acceptance and empathy which the therapist experiences for [them]" (Rogers, 1957, p. 99). At some level, clients tend to reciprocally communicate that they have received the therapist's attempts at UPR and empathic attunement—even subtly, sometimes verbally, and often non-verbally. This condition captures the reciprocal nature of feeling, being, and communicating in humanistic psychotherapy.

Dialogue and Inclusion

Because humanistic sandtray therapists avoid forcing anything on the client and instead provide a space for what is happening to emerge and be explored, HST incorporates two keystones of gestalt theory related to the therapeutic relationship: dialogue and inclusion. *Dialogue* is "what emerges when you and I come together in an authentically contactful manner" (Yontef, 1993, p. 39). Dialogue is not a condition into which humanistic sandtray therapists put effort. Instead, dialogic contact happens when humanistic sandtray therapists prepare to bring their "will to the boundary" (p. 40) and gracefully allow for the client to respond.

Inclusion is a fundamental gestalt-oriented concept that is one of the ventricles of the heart of the therapeutic relationship. Yontef (1993) defined inclusion as

> Feeling into the other's view while maintaining the sense of yourself. The person practicing inclusion sees the world for a moment as fully

as possible through the other's eyes. And it is not confluent, since the person practicing inclusion simultaneously maintains a sense of themselves as a separate person. It is the highest form of polar awareness of self and other. (p. 36)

Furthermore, Yontef differentiated inclusion from empathy: "Inclusion includes moving further into the pole of feeling the other's viewpoint than is sometimes meant by the term empathy, while simultaneously keeping a sharper awareness of one's separate existence than is sometimes implied in the term empathy" (p. 36).

In HST, I consider inclusion a particularly deep form of contact and dialogue with clients. Because sandtray work exposes clients to a kind of psychological nakedness, humanistic sandtray therapists must allow themselves to connect with what emerges between client and therapist from the client's point of view. Inclusion captures the profound depth of this relationship couched in realness that can ignite when a client creates and processes their sandtray scene.

The Experiential Nature of Learning and Change

When humanistic sandtray therapists work with a client and their sandtray, they accept who the client is and how they are experiencing and making contact. The flow of contact in an HST session can turn toward the therapeutic relationship, miniatures in the sandtray, the tray as a whole, the client's emergent emotions, their physiological experience, or their memories, for example. Because the nature of learning and change in humanistic therapy is experiential, the humanistic sandtray therapist's goal is to invite the client into increased awareness moment-to- moment. Although the client is in the lead, the therapist acts as facilitator and a guide into the here and now. At times, the therapist may be in a mostly non-directive stance, and other times they may be more directive.

Awareness versus Insight

HST focuses on "*what* clients are experiencing and *how* they experience it [rather] than why" (Armstrong et al., 2017, p. 221; italics theirs). What and how refer to awareness, and why refers to insight. HST is not an insight-oriented approach (Armstrong, 2008), although some clients do gain new understandings of the origins of their dysfunctional patterns, and that insight can be very important to them. In HST, change is rooted in experiencing fully what emerges for the client, particularly in terms of their physio-emotional awareness. When I train therapists in HST, I like to tell them that a major goal is to assist clients in moving from their heads to their hearts. Focusing on awareness is simple but not at all easy.

Rohr (1999) observed that people tend to become anxious when entering into awareness. Awareness can be uncomfortable and unsettling. It can feel threatening to people. Even in a good therapeutic environment, awareness can *feel* unsafe to clients. Many clients have very little background history with awareness, and sitting with their emotional experiences places them in a vulnerable position that may remind them of other times that they have been vulnerable, even though there is no objective threat involved during sandtray therapy. Awareness work requires the therapist to be patient, gentle, warm, and open—both with the client and with themselves.

Unless the therapist or client owns a DeLorean that can go 88 miles per hour and generate the 1.21 gigawatts necessary for time travel, neither party involved in humanistic sandtray therapy can change the past or the future. What a client can change, if they so choose, is the immediate present. With increased awareness, clients can see more clearly their choices regarding how to feel, how and what to perceive, or how to respond or act. Carson (2003) called this position being *at choice*. In HST, being at choice does not mean "developing new *shoulds*" (p. 110; italics theirs). Being at choice means experiencing awareness that assists the client with clarity about all the many decisions they can make moment to moment. Awareness is fundamental to client change because of its basis in the paradoxical theory of change (Beisser, 1970).

Paradoxical Theory of Change

Humanistic sandtray therapists operate under the philosophical assumption that given a safe and trusting therapeutic relationship, lasting therapeutic change is rooted fundamentally in the paradoxical theory of change: "*change occurs when one becomes what [one] is, not when [one] tries to become what [one] is not*" (Beisser, 1970, p. 77, italics theirs). In HST, therapists do not force clients to change. Humanistic sandtray therapists co-create an environment in psychotherapy that allows clients to be where, who, how, and what they are. By discovering who they fully are and how they are experiencing in the here and now, clients are brought at choice and can opt (or not) to change. The most important part of the work here is that clients experience fully who they are underneath all their defenses, shoulds, and perceptions. When clients can be present with who they really are—warts and all—then they feel a sense of freedom and choice. HST provides an effective medium by which clients can be invited into this process.

Qualities of Effective Humanistic Sandtray Therapists

Homeyer and Lyles (2022) emphasized the importance of the person of the sandtray therapist. Based on my experience training and supervising psychotherapists in HST, I wholeheartedly agree that who the humanistic sandtray therapist is as a person impacts significantly their ability to facilitate healing alongside their clients. Many thought leaders in the fields of psychotherapy and counseling have remarked on characteristics that make for an effective humanistic therapist (e.g., Rogers, 1951; Yalom, 1980; Yontef, 1993; Zinker, 1977). Here I review qualities of therapists that impact provision of effective humanistic sandtray therapy.

- *Humanistic sandtray therapists have "walked the walk" in psychotherapy.* They have attended their own personal psychotherapy and return to do more work when they sense internal disruption. They create intentional opportunities for self-growth, resolution of their unfinished business, and increased self-awareness.
- *Humanistic sandtray therapists are invested in their organismic self-regulation.* In order to engage in presence, empathic attunement, inclusion, and contact, therapists must engage in their own sense of living and being, both outside and inside of the consultation room. They have integrated a practice of good contact and have learned how to connect with supportive material and withdraw from toxic material. This allows them to bring their experiences of good contact into the therapeutic relationship.
- *Humanistic sandtray therapists have significant experience creating their own sandtrays.* Investment in creation of their own trays allows therapists to experience the process on both sides of the tray. It is important that they immerse themselves in the power of humanistic sandtray therapy as creators. Not only can it lead to the therapists' healing, but also it provides greater access to empathy with their clients.
- *Humanistic sandtray therapists invest in the power of vulnerability and openness.* Sandtray work has potential to be a vulnerable process for client and therapist. Therapists need to have good boundaries, which means that they know where to arrive in terms of the contact boundary permeability–impermeability continuum to best reach their clients moment to moment.
- *Humanistic sandtray therapists are attuned to microawareness.* Yontef (1993) described microawareness as awareness of the awareness process. Therapists allow themselves to simply notice (Carson, 2003) what emerges for them and how their process of emergence is taking place.

HST is a system of psychotherapy that can open new opportunities for discovery for clients and their therapists. It can be a profound experience within the dialogic relationship filled with presence, authenticity, and awareness. When therapists dedicate themselves to the craft of HST, they uncover new avenues for living within themselves and their clients.

Conclusion

HST is a theoretical model of sandtray therapy that is based on person-centered gestalt tenets. In this model, humanistic sandtray therapists integrate a method of care that exposes clients to a multisensory, indirect, and cathartic therapeutic experience. Humanistic sandtray therapists emphasize the real relationship, awareness, and paradox as drivers of client change in psychotherapy and believe that the process of HST can be a powerful medium through which deep healing takes place.

References

Allan, J., & Berry, P. (1987). Sandplay. *Elementary School Guidance & Counseling*, *21*(4), 300–306.

Armstrong, S. A. (2008). *Sandtray therapy: A humanistic approach*. Ludic Press.

Armstrong, S. A., Foster, R. D., Brown, T., & Davis, J. (2017). Humanistic sandtray therapy with children and adults. In E. S. Leggett & J. N. Boswell (Eds.), *Directive play therapy: Theories and techniques* (pp. 217–253). Springer.

Beisser, A. (1970). The paradoxical theory of change. In J. Fagan & I. L. Shepherd (Eds.), *Gestalt therapy now: Theories, techniques, applications* (pp. 77–80). Science and Behavior Books.

Boik, B. L., & Goodwin, E. A. (2000). *Sandplay therapy: A step-by-step manual for psychotherapists of diverse orientations*. W. W. Norton & Co.

Bradway, K. (1996). Sandplay and sandtray. *Journal of Sandplay Therapy, 5*(2), 9–11.

Bradway, K. (2002). Response to Clifford Mayes and Pamela Backwell-Mayes paper: The use of sandplay in a graduate educational leadership program. *Journal of Sandplay Therapy, 11*(2), 103.

Bradway, K. (2006). What is sandplay? *Journal of Sandplay Therapy, 15*(2), 7–10.

Cain, D. J. (2002). Defining characteristics, history, and evolution of humanistic psychotherapies. In D. J. Cain & J. Seeman (Eds.), *Humanistic psychotherapies: Handbook of research and practice* (pp. 3–54). American Psychological Association.

Carson, R. (2003). *Taming your gremlin: A surprisingly simple method for getting out of your own way* (Revised ed.). William Morrow.

Dawson, P. H. (2024). *Sand therapy for out of control sexual behavior, shame, and trauma: Treatment approaches beyond words*. Routledge.

Day, R., & Day, C. (2012). *Creative therapy in the sand*. Brook Creative Therapy.

Fall, K. A., Holden, J. M., & Marquis, A. (2023). *Theoretical models of counseling and psychotherapy* (4th ed.). Routledge. https://doi.org/10.4324/9781000 3189770

Fleet, D. (2023). *Pluralistic sand-tray therapy: Humanistic principles for working creatively with adult clients*. Routledge. https://doi.org/10.4324/9781000 3158707

Frank, J. D., & Frank, J. B. (1991). *Persuasion and healing: A comparative study of psychotherapy* (3rd ed.). The Johns Hopkins University Press.

Herlihy, B. (1985). Person-centered gestalt therapy: A synthesis. *Journal of Humanistic Education and Development, 24*(1), 16–24. https://doi.org/10.1002/j.2164-4683.1985.tb00274.x

Homeyer, L. E., & Lyles, M. N. (2022). *Advanced sandtray therapy: Digging deeper into clinical practice*. Routledge. https://doi.org/10.4324/9781003095491

Homeyer, L. E., & Sweeney, D. S. (2023). *Sandtray therapy: A practical manual* (4th ed.). Routledge. https://doi.org/10.4324/9781003221418

Kalff, D. (1971). *Sandplay: Mirror of a child's psyche*. C. G. Jung Institute.

Kottman, T. (2023). Adlerian applications of sandtray play therapy. *World Journal for Sand Therapy Practice, 1*(3). https://doi.org/10.58997/wjstp.v1i3.17

Landreth, G. L. (2023). *Play therapy: The art of the relationship* (4th ed.). Routledge. https://doi.org/10.4324/9781003255796

Lewin, K. (1951). *Field theory in social science: Selected theoretical papers*. Harper & Brothers.

Lowenfeld, M. (1950). The nature and use of the Lowenfeld World Technique in work with children and adults. *The Journal of Psychology, 30*, 325–331. https://doi.org/10.1080/00223980.1950.9916070

Lowenfeld, M. (2007). *Understanding children's sandplay: Lowenfeld's World Technique*. Sussex Academic Press.

Mann, D. (2021). *Gestalt therapy: 100 key points and techniques* (2nd ed.). Routledge. https://doi.org/10.4324/9781315158495

Parlett, M. (1991). Reflections on field theory. *British Gestalt Journal, 1*(2), 69–81.

Pearson, M., & Wilson, H. (2009). *Using expressive arts to work with mind, body and emotions*. Jessica Kingsley.

Perls, F. S. (1959). *Gestalt therapy verbatim*. Real People Press.

Perls, F., Hefferline, R., & Goodman, P. (1951/1994). *Gestalt therapy: Excitement and growth in the human personality*. The Gestalt Journal Press.

Polster, E., & Polster, M. (1973). *Gestalt therapy integrated: Contours of theory & practice*. Brunner/Mazel.

Preston-Dillon, D. (2009, March). Narrative approaches in sand therapy: Transformative journeys for counselor and client. Paper based on a program presented at the American Counseling Association Annual Conference and Exposition, Charlotte, NC. *VISTAS Online*.

Rogers, C. R. (1942). *Counseling and psychotherapy: Newer concepts in practice*. Houghton Mifflin.

Rogers, C. R. (1951). *Client-centered therapy: Its current practice, implications and theory*. Houghton-Mifflin.

Rogers, C. R. (1957). The necessary and sufficient conditions of therapeutic personality change. *Journal of Consulting Psychology, 21*(2), 95–103. https://psycnet.apa.org/doi/10.1037/h0045357

Rogers, C. R. (1959). A theory of therapy, personality, and inter-personal relationships, as developed in the client-centered framework. In S. Koch (Ed.), *Psychology: A study of a science. Formulations of the person and social context. Vol. 3*. McGraw-Hill.

Rogers, C. R. (1989). A client-centered/person-centered approach to therapy. In H. Kirschenbaum & V. L. Henderson (Eds.), *The Carl Rogers reader* (pp. 135–156). Houghton Mifflin.

Rohr, R. (1999). *Everything belongs: The gift of contemplative prayer.* Crossroad Publishing.

Smith, S. D. (2012). *Sandtray play and storymaking: A hands-on approach to build academic, social, and emotional skills in mainstream and special education.* Jessica Kingsley.

Wampold, B. E., & Imel, Z. E. (2015). *The great psychotherapy debate: The evidence for what makes psychotherapy work* (2nd ed.). Routledge. https://doi.org/10.4324/9780203582015

Wilkins, P. (2016). *Person-centred therapy: 100 key points & techniques* (2nd ed.). Routledge. https://doi.org/10.4324/9781315765198

Yalom, I. D. (1980). *Existential psychotherapy.* Basic Books.

Yontef, G. (1993). *Awareness, dialogue & process.* The Gestalt Press.

Yontef, G. (1999). Awareness, dialogue and process: Preface to the 1998 German edition. *The Gestalt Journal, 22*(1), 9–20.

Zinker, J. (1977). *Creative process in Gestalt therapy.* Brunner/Mazel.

Chapter 2

Putting Together Your Sandtray Collection and Physical Environment

Use of sandtray presents clinicians with decisions that may seem unfamiliar to them. When I first started integrating sandtray therapy into my practice while I was a doctoral student at the University of North Texas, I was privileged to work in a community counseling agency that had a sandtray therapy room. One wall was completely lined with shelves from top to bottom, left to right, with a seemingly infinite number of miniatures, carefully separated into categories. One wall had two large sandtrays filled with white-colored sand and a spray bottle to use if a client wanted to create a wet tray in order to mold the sand into mountains, valleys, hills, or other structures. It was a sandtray therapist's dream setup! When I went into private practice and started my sandtray collection from scratch, I ran into several obstacles and had to get creative. Money was probably my number one obstacle. I was familiar with Homeyer and Sweeney's (2023) detailed recommendations on everything from types of sand to categories of miniatures to trays, and immediately I wanted to get back to having a sandtray collection reflecting my deepest, nerdiest desires. However, I was lucky if I could pay my office rent every month. Therefore, I had to take a big, deep breath, center myself, and start small. I imagine many of you can identify with early sandtray therapy career limitations.

My first sandtray setup consisted of a 16-inch diameter, round sand tray for which life began as a terracotta clay plant saucer from a local hardware store. I painted the bottom and sides a medium blue to represent water and sky, as Homeyer and Sweeney (2023) suggested, and filled the tray with all-natural, non-toxic white sand. I added wheels to the legs of an old round end table I had that just happened to be the same circumference as the bottom of my sand tray and used it to prop the tray up. I had no shelves, but I had a card table that I placed the figures on, out in the open of my private practice office. I had maybe 35 miniatures. I began to shop at dollar stores and garage sales, and rummaged through my old toys that my parents had been holding on to since I moved out of their house over a decade prior. After a couple of years, I added a small shelf for the

DOI: 10.4324/9781032664996-3

figures. Eventually, I outgrew the shelf due to the number of miniatures I purchased over time.

I learned several lessons by having to start from scratch. I learned about my resourcefulness. I learned that clients' scenes could be limited by the materials available—the size of the tray, the number and types of miniatures, for example—and that these limitations are not inherently bad for client work. I learned that even a single sandtray figure could change the course of a client's therapeutic work. I also learned, to be cliché, that every sandtray therapist starts somewhere and that I had a habit of applying shoulds to myself along the way (e.g., I should have an expansive and admirable sandtray collection; otherwise, my clients will not benefit, and I will be the laughingstock of the sandtray therapy world). When I train therapists in HST, I encourage them to get started with intention in context of reality. The physical components to sandtray therapy do matter, but clients have creatively endured their own unfinished business, so certainly they can engage in that same creative energy within a sandtray setup that diverges from perfection.

Fast forward to now, and I have a close-to-ideal setup. I *finally* purchased a standard-sized tray—a rectangular shape, approximately 28.5 inches long × 19.5 inches wide × 3 inches deep, complete with a detachable rolling cart designed just for the tray. I have my dream shelf setup of tall shelves that I have filled up yet again, and as I type this sentence, I am thinking of adding another. I still do not have all the miniatures I want—but ask any sandtray therapist and I think we have all turned buying figures into a bit of an obsession. I continually discover what I do not have when clients are building a scene and looking for a miniature that captures their metaphor just right. I have settled into believing that my miniatures collection will be a lifelong incomplete gestalt. A humanistic sandtray therapist's sandtray collection will never be perfect because of the idiosyncrasy of each clinician's work setting, population, office space requirements, and preferences. However, I encourage you to invest intentionally in your decision-making. I highly recommend that every sandtray therapist read Homeyer and Sweeney's (2023) detailed discussion about these matters as a companion to this chapter. My aim is to provide guidance for creating a sandtray setup that is based on humanistic philosophy, client population needs, clinical setting, physical space issues, and therapist creativity. Moreover, I discuss telehealth sandtray in this chapter.

The Sand Tray

The sand tray acts as an environment in which the client and counselor allow dialogic contact to emerge. Its solid walls and foundation are impermeable and, therefore, structured with a bottom and four sides, yet it maintains some permeability because it is accessible from above. Homeyer and Sweeney (2023) referred to the tray as a "sacred space" (p. 27); therefore, you should be purposeful about selecting the size and kind of tray that you use. Although what the sandtray community labels as a standard-sized tray grew out of Dora Kalff's recommendation and approximates 30 inches × 20 inches × 3 inches, I encourage you to experiment with different sizes or shapes if they better fit the client needs, physical environment, or nature of the therapist's job. Following are some issues you should consider:

- In terms of tray size, I echo Homeyer and Sweeney's (2023) conceptualization of the sand tray as representative of a gestalt; therefore, an ability to view the entire tray from a single vantage point is important in HST. Although clients may at various times focus on different parts of their sandtray scene, in keeping with humanistic philosophy, the therapist needs to make room for the holistic nature of the metaphor.
- Some tray shapes may be more conducive to group sandtray (see Chapter 9). For example, when I was a graduate student learning sandtray from Linda Homeyer, we worked in an octagonal tray in groups of four. This setup gave me enough room to navigate as much of the tray as I wanted without violating other group members' physical space. The tray allowed for good contact between the tray, group members, and me.
- Some clinicians may need to use a portable sand tray if they are doing in-home work, traveling between schools, or have shared office spaces. When I did some traveling sandtray work, I used a blue-tinted, casserole-sized plastic food storage container with a lid so the sand did not spill out. I have also used small portable trays that can be purchased online easily. However, therapists can purchase full-size portable plastic trays with lids, as well.

In Parts II and III, I will provide specific guidance regarding trays appropriate for a variety of populations and clinical settings.

The Miniatures

Sandtray miniatures form the ground in the figure–ground relationship, and the client's emerging awareness in the moment, such as their reaction to an element of the scene, is the figure. Miniatures and the way they are arranged in the tray are metaphors for the client's perceptions of self, others, memories, attachments, dreams, hopes, emotions, and shoulds. Because ground has a limitless quality to it, providing access to as many symbols as possible is an important consideration for humanistic sandtray therapists. In HST, I encourage therapists to use Homeyer and Sweeney's (2023) guide to building a miniatures collection. They provide a checklist for a basic set consisting of 300 miniatures categorized by type. Of course, this would be reasonable for a therapist who is in a permanent office, but I encourage you to be flexible with the number of miniatures. In a beginning collection, I strongly recommend the following:

- Have a variety of figures across Homeyer and Sweeney's categories, rather than focusing on the 300 miniatures minimum.
- Ensure the therapist provides access to miniatures that are designed for their client population. In this text, I review specific guidance for miniatures representative of populations in Parts II and III.
- Include objects that can represent the actualizing tendency, growth, and completion of the gestalt, such as bridges, butterflies and caterpillars, rainbows, and plants (both flowering and non-flowering).
- Provide a variety of miniatures that represent boundaries across the impermeable and permeable continuum. For example, include different kinds of fences (solid and porous), stone and brick walls, doors, and windows.
- Focus on having opposites included in your miniature collection to reflect the gestalt concepts of paradox and contact boundary disturbances, such as sun and moon, heroes and villains, babies and adults (humans and animals), fire and water, and so on.

Although lists and categories of figures can be helpful to the beginning humanistic sandtray therapist, I recommend that therapists follow their instincts and their sense of what could be useful to clients. When sandtray therapists attend to their awareness in practical matters, they may find, like I have, that their intuitive sense can lead them to choose figures that may not have a logical connection to a current client or population. However, I have witnessed clients use newly purchased miniatures that I did not fathom they would use, and during the process I felt deep contact emerge.

Another issue regarding miniatures is storage and display. When a clinician is privileged enough to have their own consultation room in which they keep a permanent sandtray collection, then an ideal setup is open shelves on which miniatures are displayed at a height most comfortable for the client population (Homeyer & Sweeney, 2023). In shared permanent spaces, therapists may want to mount a curtain on the shelves or purchase shelves with solid doors. When I have counseling interns doing sandtray in middle schools, they utilize a shelf on wheels with miniatures kept in lidless plastic containers from the dollar store. For therapists who travel for in-home counseling or within school districts, I recommend a duffle bag that stores a portable tray and plastic fishing lure containers. My friend and co-developer of HST, Steve Armstrong, used fishing tackle boxes because he traveled for his sandtray trainings. There are many other ways of storing and displaying miniatures, and it is something about which I encourage you to think intently.

The Physical Environment

In addition to sand trays and miniatures, the physical environment in which HST takes place is integral to clients' experiences. The physical psychotherapy environment can impact the client's immediate experiencing of safety and openness (Meier & Davis, 2019) and, if it is a space that is controlled by the therapist, communicates something about the therapist to the client. Major elements to attend to are the room setup and furniture.

Room Setup and Furniture

Armstrong (2008) stated that "[w]hen clients come into my private practice office, I want them to feel like they are entering a safe haven" (p. 64). The room in which therapist and client meet for HST should be large enough to accommodate shelving (or other ways of storing miniatures), miniatures, the sand tray, and therapist and client seats. The client should be able to move freely 360 degrees around the sand tray as they create their scene. I recommend that the therapist and client have a triangular relationship to the sand tray (see Figure 2.1). Sitting in this manner allows them to face each other without a psychological obstacle and allows the therapist to see the tray from as close to the client's point of view as possible.

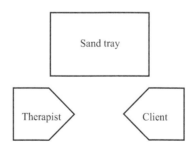

Figure 2.1 Therapist and client triangular relationship to the sand tray.

Finally, ensure that the client and therapist can fully see the tray without straining by making sure the tray's height is between the client's abdomen and shoulders. A sand tray that is too low may mean client and therapist are arching their backs, creating unnecessary physiological tension. Some clients prefer sitting on the floor, so in that case, sit on the floor with them and place the tray on the floor, too.

Digital Sandtray

Distance counseling online was a niche area of practice before 2020 (Williamson & Williamson, 2021). Mental health practitioners witnessed their professional worlds change dramatically as they shifted to telehealth practice during the COVID-19 pandemic. After the initial jolt, they began seeking out ways to integrate typical in-person approaches to a virtual environment. Although at least one digital sandtray platform existed before the COVID-19 pandemic, based on my anecdotal experience, they certainly became more widely used when clinicians implemented social distancing parameters in their professional lives. I begin by discussing a few major platforms that offer digital sandtray therapy and conclude by discussing the impact of digital sandtray platforms on HST.

Platforms

Currently, there are three major platforms that offer access to digital sandtray: Virtual Sandtray® (2020b), Simply Sand Play (n.d.), and Online Sand Tray (Fried, 2023). All of them share basic similarities: a graphical interface in which a sandtray is visible and a selection of digital miniatures. Users can manipulate the placement, size, and direction of the miniatures. On each platform, the user can save a picture of the sandtray scene that they have created, and one option is for the therapist to direct their client to share the saved image file of their sandtray scene via a HIPAA HITECH (U.S. Department of Health and Human Services, 2017) compatible platform. However, with the advent of screen share over many telehealth platforms, it is possible for the therapist to observe the client's process of scene construction. Two of the platforms, Virtual Sandtray and Simply Sand Play, are free for clients but therapists pay for access. Online Sand Tray is freely accessible to anyone.

VSA is a partner of the Dr. Margaret Lowenfeld Trust and was an early pioneer of digital sandtray. Initially, the developer of VSA designed it for use face-to-face with clients (Kaduson, 2022). They offer over 7,000 models, which is their term for miniatures (Virtual Sandtray, 2020a). Simply Sand Play offers thousands of miniatures as well (M. Georgieva, 2022, personal communication). These platforms are similar in that they integrate a three-dimensional interface, allow users to change details of miniatures such as the color of skin or hair on human miniatures, and provide users choices in terms of what color of sand they use. In addition, the vantage point can be changed to view the scene from any angle, and users can zoom into parts of the tray on which they want to focus. Online Sand Tray differs from the other two platforms in that it is a two-dimensional, top-down view. The selection of miniatures is more limited than the other platforms but offers, in my opinion, a good variety.

Impact of Digital Sandtray on HST

Improving telehealth access to mental health care is critical for clients who have difficulty engaging in traditional counseling and psychotherapy (Williamson & Williamson, 2021). Clients with limited incomes may have transportation issues. Clients from rural areas may have very few options in terms of mental health care providers in their areas. A potential obstacle particular to traditional in-person sandtray therapy for some clients may be due to ability differences, such as sensitivity to the sand and/or the miniatures. Certainly, digital sandtray can provide access to the power of this approach to clients who have challenging or limited access to traditional in-person HST.

Whereas there are many potential advantages for clients when therapists use digital sandtray platforms, there are also some important considerations that appear to limit the power of HST. First, and perhaps most obvious, is the lack of a kinesthetic component. A major part of humanistic therapy involves engaging all senses available to a client, and there can be ways of adapting traditional in-person HST for clients who are sensitive to touch, such as people who are neurodiverse, without resorting to a platform that completely removes clients from a connection with their bodies, the miniatures, and the sand (see Chapter 8). Second, as much as digital sandtray platforms can be visually engaging, the two platforms that are three-dimensional in nature are perceptual tricks. Clients can maintain a sense of distance from the computer screen because of the unreality of the scenes and trays. Real miniatures and a real tray are unmistakable and bring a presence into the room that is difficult to do virtually. Third, navigating through the various miniatures or models in a virtual platform can be tedious. Anecdotally, some of my supervisees have "settled for" miniatures out of a sense of giving up because they get tired of scrolling. Although there are search functions, clients cannot see all the figures in front of them as they can with in-person sandtray.

Finally, I wonder if digital sandtray platforms are really sandtray at all. There is no sand, there is no tray, and there are no miniatures—only depictions of these elements. They are approximations of sandtray. Homeyer and Sweeney (2023) posited that newer approaches that developers label as sand therapy may not be sandtray equivalent, but they also may not have to be. Like many of the decisions humanistic sandtray therapists must make that I have outlined in this chapter, I encourage you to consider wisely use of a digital sandtray platform by weighing strengths and limitations for your individual clients. Psychotherapy approaches are not one-size-fits-all and it may be that some benefits outweigh the limitations of digital sandtray for clients who have challenges engaging in traditional sandtray work, whether in-person or via telehealth.

Conclusion

Humanistic sandtray therapists have many decisions to make as they are building their sandtray collection of miniatures and trays. I strongly encourage you to allow your clients, clinical setting, and pocketbook to guide you as you curate your miniatures over time. In addition, I recommend that you set up your counseling space thoughtfully with depth of connection and the therapeutic relationship in mind, including your consideration of using a virtual sandtray platform. Building a full sandtray collection takes a lot of time, effort, and money, and it can be challenging and fun. I feel my creative spirit when I choose new miniatures that I think would work well with certain clients, and I hope that you experience similar sensations as you start or continue your collection.

References

Armstrong, S. A. (2008). *Sandtray therapy: A humanistic approach*. Ludic Press.

Fried, K. (2023). Online sand tray. https://www.onlinesandtray.com/

Homeyer, L. E., & Sweeney, D. S. (2023). *Sandtray therapy: A practical manual* (4th ed.). Routledge.

Kaduson, H. G. (2022). Using the Virtual Sandtray® app: A boy's journey to healing. In J. Stone (Ed.), *Play therapy and telemental health* (pp. 173–186). Routledge. https://doi.org/10.4324/9781003166498-11

Meier, S. T., & Davis, S. R. (2019). *The elements of counseling* (8th ed.). Waveland Press.

Simply Sand Play. (n.d.). Simply Sand Play. https://simplysandplay.com/

U.S. Department of Health and Human Services. (2017). HITECH Act Enforcement Interim Final Rule. https://www.hhs.gov/hipaa/for-profession als/special-topics/hitech-act-enforcement-interim-final-rule/index.html

Virtual Sandtray. (2020a). Models. https://www.virtualsandtray.org/models

Virtual Sandtray (2020b). Virtual Sandtray homepage. https://www.virtualsandt ray.org/

Williamson, J. N., & Williamson, D. G. (2021). Preface. In J. N. Williamson & D. G. Williamson (Eds.), *Distance counseling and supervision: A guide for mental health clinicians* (pp. vii–viii). American Counseling Association.

Chapter 3

Structure and Phases of Humanistic Sandtray Therapy

HST is considered an experiment in psychotherapy. It has an underlying structure formed by phases that generally follow Homeyer and Sweeney's (2023) stepwise process. Each phase requires the humanistic sandtray therapist's active facilitation; in HST, therapists facilitate the process and clients provide the content of therapy. Although humanistic sandtray therapists generally follow the client's lead (Armstrong, 2008), the therapist should attend to their observations to know when to transition to the next HST phase. For clients who are new to sandtray therapy, the therapist may be more directive in moving toward the next phase. However, I have noticed that with my clients who have done multiple sandtrays, they tend to build an intuitive sense that moves them forward through the process. Pernet and Caplin (2022) described the sandtray process in terms of the gestalt cycle of experience (Zinker, 1977). They conceptualized seven stages of a single sandtray session. In HST, I conceptualize sandtray sessions as having five phases. Following I will describe the five phases of HST and integrate them with Pernet and Caplin's (2022) process view of sandtray.

Pre-creation Phase

The *pre-creation phase* captures the client's vague sensory-emotional experience and the beginning of clarity of the emerging figure in the figure/ground relationship. Prior to the client and therapist discussing the notion of sandtray, the client enters the sensation phase in the gestalt cycle of experience (Pernet & Caplin, 2022). They feel or sense the unclear edges of a memory, image, feeling, or physical sensation. Next, the client makes initial contact with the sand tray and miniatures. This contact may be initiated by the therapist or the client; however, in either case, contact is based on the client's emerging experience, aligning with the awareness stage in the gestalt cycle of experience (Pernet & Caplin, 2022). The client begins to experience more clearly a sensory, emotional, or cognitive response that links them with a potential for sandtray work.

DOI: 10.4324/9781032664996-4

In the case of the therapist initiating sandtray work, sometimes they will introduce the client to a general description of sandtray a session or two before the client creates their tray if the therapist believes sandtray might be a good fit. My typical introduction to sandtray goes something like:

> I wanted to direct your attention to the shelves full of miniature figures over in the corner and that tray of white sand. Those items are part of an approach I sometimes use with clients called sandtray. Sandtray is a way to create a scene that captures what clients want to communicate in therapy but may have a difficult time doing for a variety of reasons. If you're curious to experiment with sandtray, I think it could be a good fit for you.

This approach is generally applicable with older adolescents and adults. For pre-adolescents and young adolescents, I prefer not to prepare them ahead of time, as this can increase their already strong defenses; I tend to invite them into sandtray work spontaneously. Another way I introduce sandtray to clients is through use of the miniatures only. For example, I asked one of my female clients who had a particularly low self-concept to pick a miniature that seemed to beckon her. I requested that she not think too much about it. She had never created a sandtray scene. She picked an Eeyore miniature, and I asked her to describe Eeyore to me. She stated that he was droopy, gloomy, and always lost his tail. She began to tear up and I asked her, "What is coming up for you with your tears?" She expressed to me, "Oh my god! *I'm* Eeyore!" In that moment, I could tell she felt intense contact with the miniature. My client's here-and-now experiencing of Eeyore as she described him led her into the mobilization stage of the gestalt cycle of experience (Pernet & Caplin, 2022). Seeing herself as Eeyore led to development of a figure in which her need for self-acceptance arose. Her experience led her into microawareness and changed the course of her psychotherapy because she was able to be more honest with herself and with me. Eeyore was present in the therapy room as it often arose as my client's figure, indicating a need emerging, until our termination session many months later.

When the client initiates contact, it often comes in the form of curiosity. They may ask questions about the tray or the miniatures. In those moments, typically I invite them to check out the miniatures and experience the sand. Many times, the client will run their hands and fingers through the sand and may have a notable response: some clients feel soothed by the sand, whereas others may feel disgust and draw away their hand. The client's response to the sand and their response to the miniatures are important non-verbals for you to observe. They may indicate the client's readiness to move toward the creation phase.

The pre-creation phase can differ widely depending on the client's past experiences with sandtray. For example, clients who are new to sandtray may want to spend more time exploring the miniatures and encountering the sand and to connect their inner experiencing with the potential for symbolization. These clients may re-enter the pre-creation phase at the beginning of the next session. Over time, when a client creates multiple scenes, the pre-creation phase may consist of sensation(s) arising within the client who then indicates they are ready to move into the creation phase.

Creation Phase

The beginning of the creation phase in HST correlates with the awareness, mobilization, and action stages of the gestalt cycle of experience (Pernet & Caplin, 2022). I begin with a short centering exercise in which I guide my client into the present moment and focus on their breathing. My objective with centering is to emphasize the awareness stage and to bring the figure and need into increased clarity for the client. Centering lasts about two minutes. Following is a centering exercise that I use:

> Before we start the sandtray process, let's take a few moments to center ourselves. As we center, some people prefer to close their eyes and others prefer to leave them open. If you leave your eyes open, find something in the room on which you can focus your eyes—for example, a design in the rug or a spot on the wall. Okay. What I'd like you to do is take a deep breath in, filling up your lungs like a balloon, then exhale all your air as if you're deflating that balloon. As you breathe in, your tummy should extend outwards, and as you breathe out, your tummy should collapse.
>
> Go ahead and keep taking these deep, long breaths. As you close your eyes (or focus on an object in the room), check out each part of your body, starting from your toes. Check your toes out, then move up your legs past your knees, up to your stomach and chest. Spend a little bit of time in each part of your body. If you get distracted by a thought or a sound, return to your breath and focus there. Keep checking out your body's sensations, from your chest out to your shoulders, arms, hands, and fingers. Then back to your chest, up your neck, your face, and your head.
>
> Return to your breathing and keep your awareness there. Notice how your breath passes through your nose and into your lungs and out. Now place your awareness on your eyelids. Notice how heavy they feel. When

you are ready, slowly open your eyes, allowing your eyelids to float up like a cloud. Come back to the room.

The mobilization stage starts with a sandtray prompt. For an older adolescent or adult client who is creating their first sandtray, the typical HST prompt follows (Armstrong, personal communication, 2011):

> What I would like you to do is create a scene of your life the way it is now. You may include elements from the past or future but focus mainly on how your life is presently. I want you to be brutally honest with yourself as you create your scene. What you choose to share with me is up to you.

For preadolescents and young adolescents, a more directive prompt is appropriate. For example, the therapist may state: "I'd like you to make a scene in the tray about your life at school." Additionally, Homeyer and Lyles (2022) and Homeyer and Sweeney (2023) provided multiple example prompts that work well in HST. Philosophically, good sandtray prompts respond to the client's here-and-now emotion, sensation, image, or thought.

As the client makes their sandtray scene, they enter the action stage of the gestalt cycle of experience (Pernet & Caplin, 2022). Often, I play soft background music at a low volume. If the therapist chooses to play music, it should be wordless and as neutral as possible. Generally, the therapist should remain quiet during scene creation. Sometimes the client will talk to me while they select miniatures and arrange their scene. I generally respond with minimal encouragers, such as, "Hmm," or a quiet head nod. In HST, the therapist attunes to their observational skills of the client's creation process. You should not only carefully attend to the client's construction of the tray—such as where they place miniatures in relation to each other, miniatures they pick up and put back or spend a long time thinking about using, or how they rearrange the scene—but also any emotions that arise. The creation phase can hold therapeutic power for the client and bring their emotions to the surface. I have witnessed deep pain emerge during this phase as clients become tearful or even angry. Noticing what comes up for the client will indicate how to begin the processing phase.

Processing Phase

The *processing phase* of HST aligns with the action and contact phases of the gestalt cycle of experience (Pernet & Caplin, 2022). If the client appears to be experiencing something at the beginning of the processing phase, I typically reflect the client's feelings or non-verbals and may ask a discovery-oriented question. For example, if a client is tearful as they indicate they are finished creating their tray, I might say, "You seem to be experiencing something quite powerful. What's it like to feel your tears?" If I cannot quite tell what a client is experiencing as we enter the processing phase, then I might say, "What is it like to create your scene?" Because the emphasis in HST is on immediate experiencing and awareness, I recommend starting with a reflection or question that is likely to spark exploration of the here and now. However, if the client appears to be reflective but somewhat neutral, I might begin with, "Tell me about your scene." Follow your client's lead. Because the processing phase is where skillful HST work takes place, I discuss explicitly the therapist's roles in these mechanics as well as client dynamics that may emerge in Chapter 4.

Post-creation Phase

During the post-creation phase of HST, the client and therapist have exited the focused sandtray experience and are processing the process. This phase corresponds to the satisfaction stage of the gestalt cycle of experience (Pernet & Caplin, 2022). The post-creation phase encapsulates not only the immediate remainder of the session in which the client engaged in sandtray, but also often carries on into future sessions. The satisfaction stage is likely to carry on in future sessions as clients work through and reflect on their experiences that emerged as a result of sandtray. Immediately following the HST processing phase, the therapist and client reflect on the sandtray experience. Sometimes, they may sit in relative quiet as the therapeutic post-creation space can be heavy with new figures emerging from ground. It may be that the ground has even shifted a bit for both client and therapist. If I sense a client is open to verbal dialogue, it is typical in HST for me to ask, "What's coming up for you right now as you sit in the space between your sandtray experience and ending the session?" When I train therapists in HST, I often relate to them the importance of allowing the client to have their experience. Sometimes therapists want to make sure the client is "okay" before they terminate the session. However, in HST, therapists value clients' immediate experiencing and awareness, no matter how painful. Therefore, you should avoid getting into a fix-it mode to try to make the client "feel better." Of course, there is a stark difference between a client leaving the session with suicidal ideation or in a crisis mode versus clients who have become aware of significant hurt and feel jostled, and you should use appropriate crisis management approaches if warranted.

Clean-Up Phase

The clean-up phase in HST is brief as the client is in the withdrawal stage of the gestalt cycle of experience (Pernet & Caplin, 2022). The client is invited to take a picture of the tray. Many clients will continue to process their sandtray experience between therapy sessions and it is likely that the scene, its metaphors, and the client's dynamic and continuing experience with their image of the scene will continue to be a topic in therapy. The session terminates and, after the client leaves, the therapist takes a picture of the tray for the client file. The HST philosophy is for the therapist to dismantle the tray after the client leaves so that the scene has an opportunity to live within the client (Armstrong, 2008; Armstrong et al., 2017; Badenoch, 2008; Pearson & Wilson, 2009).

Conclusion

Although HST is a structured approach, it provides permeability for clients to experience both safety and risk. A typical session consists of five phases, although some phases can extend beyond the session during which clients create their scenes. These phases mirror the gestalt cycle of experience and, therefore, allow humanistic sandtray therapists to remain philosophically grounded in the course of HST.

References

Armstrong, S. A. (2008). *Sandtray therapy: A humanistic approach*. Ludic Press.

Armstrong, S. A., Foster, R. D., Brown, T., & Davis, J. (2017). Humanistic sandtray therapy with children and adults. In E. S. Leggett & J. N. Boswell (Eds.), *Directive play therapy: Theories and techniques* (pp. 217–253). Springer.

Badenoch, B. (2008). *Being a brain-wise therapist: A practical guide to interpersonal neurobiology*. W. W. Norton & Company.

Homeyer, L. E., & Lyles, M. N. (2022). *Advanced sandtray therapy: Digging deeper into clinical practice*. Routledge. https://doi.org/10.4324/9781003095491

Homeyer, L. E., & Sweeney, D. S. (2023). *Sandtray therapy: A practical manual* (4th ed.). Routledge.

Pearson, M., & Wilson, H. (2009). *Using expressive arts to work with mind, body and emotions: Theory and practice*. Jessica Kingsley.

Pernet, K., & Caplin, W. (2022). The here and now of sandtray therapy: Sandtray therapy meets Gestalt therapy. In P. Cole (Ed.), *The relational heart of Gestalt therapy* (pp. 201–212). Routledge. https://doi.org/10.4324/9781003255772-19

Zinker, J. (1977). *Creative process in Gestalt therapy*. Brunner/Mazel.

Chapter 4

Process Skills and Strategies in Humanistic Sandtray Therapy

At the heart of HST is the therapeutic relationship. Once there is deep trust and safety established, then sandtray is an experiment (Stevens, 2004) worth considering for a wide range of clients. Armstrong (2008) stated that the goal of the processing phase of HST is to "*facilitate a process of exploration, expression, awareness and discovery*" (p. 75; italics his). Therefore, humanistic sandtray therapists implement psychotherapeutic skills and strategies that are intended to increase awareness. It sounds simple, but therapists are tempted often to get into a fixing mode with clients because they want to help their clients heal and no longer feel pain and hurt. Therapists would not be very good in their roles if they did not have some wish for clients to resolve their issues. However, that is not the focus of humanistic therapies in general and certainly not of HST. In this chapter, I discuss core processing skills and change strategies borne out of person-centered and gestalt theories and how therapists can apply them in the processing phase of HST.

Process and facilitative skills are intentional means by which humanistic sandtray therapists create dialogue with their clients. Because humanistic therapists believe that emotion lies at the core of awareness, HST skills focus primarily on feelings and the client's process of responding to them, which often comes in the form of concepts about self that have developed over time (Carson, 2003). Client change is paradoxical (Beisser, 1970) and a major focus is opening a space for clients to become aware of this paradox: "*I change by being fully aware of how I am*" (Armstrong, 2008, p. 76; italics his). Being fully aware of how I am means accepting myself down to the depths of my living breath, moment to moment. It means accepting my fallibility and my goodness. When clients become aware of how they are receiving nourishment or malnourishment from self and their environment or field, then they perceive more choices regarding how to participate in their own growth. In HST, therapists can assist clients in this process of increased awareness by operating in the here and now and providing facilitative, exploratory, and discovery-oriented responses. Moreover,

DOI: 10.4324/9781032664996-5

HST also provides clients and therapists with opportunity to work within the metaphor of the tray and to identify polarities and patterns of resistance.

Here and Now

When clients engage in therapy, often their expectation is to talk *about* something. They tend to stay in the "there and then." Afterall, the here and now can be painful and scary. However, the goal in HST is to help the client arrive at full awareness, and this requires therapists to use here-and-now language to shift the client's attention to the here and now. For example, imagine a client who has created a tray about their dysfunctional relationship with their partner. The client naturally begins to talk about a past event with their partner and perhaps even their feelings at the time of their experience. They use language that is couched in there and then—using the past tense. This client might say, "I felt so bad after my partner and I argued the other night." As the therapist, to bring the client into the here and now, I introduce a shift into present-tense language in my reflection of feeling: "You feel guilty as you think about that argument now." Then, the client has an opportunity to accept my invitation into their present emotions.

When clients report events or experiences, they are providing the therapist with a window to bring them into the here and now. The therapist who reflects feelings using the past tense, for example, saying, "You felt guilty," is staying in the there and then with a client, which is a cognitive mode. Bringing the client into the here and now invites clients into a feeling mode. When clients are in a there-and-then mode, whether they are focusing on the past or the future, they are likely focusing on some version of "why." They are analyzing an experience, which is one way that clients detach themselves from awareness. Humanistic sandtray therapists aim to provide the client with opportunity to form new habits of awareness by focusing on the what and how of a client's here-and-now experience. Therefore, all the skills and strategies that I discuss in this chapter are meant for therapists to couch them in the moment.

Facilitative and Exploratory Responses

Facilitative and exploratory responses are designed for the client and therapist to co-discover feelings in the moment by shifting the client's attention to here-and-now awareness. The humanistic sandtray therapist guides the client toward experiencing, staying with, and going deeper into feelings. When I work with graduate students and trainees, often they want to jump right from hearing about the client's sandtray into going as deep as possible into the client's emotion. However, I caution against this approach because it can be disruptive to the flow of a client's experience and can threaten emotional safety. Although clients may feel discomfort while entering into immediate awareness, it is usually because they are scared of their vulnerability or what they might discover about themselves (e.g., they really are as shitty as they have come to believe). Therefore, I encourage a gentle, empathic, and compassionate approach to co-navigating the client's emotional experiencing. In HST, the therapist begins with guiding the client into immediate emotion, followed by staying with emotion, and moving to going deeper into emotion. In HST, this process is called the *guiding into–staying with–going deeper cycle of emotional experiencing*. Although phase-like order sounds stepwise, it is not. Some clients are new to emotional processing and may be able to tolerate guidance into immediate emotion but feel too unsafe to move to staying with their emotion. Some clients stay with an emotion and become aware of another emotion emerging, so the therapist guides them into this newly discovered emotion. As is typical with processing in humanistic therapy, linearity is the exception rather than the rule.

Guiding into Immediate Emotion

When I discussed the importance of remaining in the here and now, I mentioned *reflecting feelings in the present tense*. This skill is basic to HST. The humanistic sandtray therapist must pair present-tense reflections of feeling with accurate empathic attunement, warmth, acceptance, and genuineness. For clients to feel safe to enter their emotional experiencing, they must sense that therapists have no agenda other than discovery and exploration. Humanistic sandtray therapists assume an active participant–observer stance, meaning that they are active participants in dialogue and contact with their client while observing their experiencing moment to moment. Remember, in HST, therapists help clients with *describing rather than analyzing their experience* and *exploring their awareness rather than solving their problem* by being fully present with the client (Armstrong, 2008).

Staying with Emotion

When clients can tolerate entering their emotional experiencing, the next step is to facilitate *staying with their emotions*. There are several ways to encourage staying with emotions. One way is the use of therapeutic silence while the therapist maintains an empathic facial expression. Another method is to invite the client to stay with their feelings: "I see your tears starting to form. Stay with your pain and notice what's coming up for you." Carson

(2003) emphasized the importance of simply noticing—being with emotional experiencing without judgment and without trying to change it.

"Staying with" is completely subjective. For a client, an especially vulnerable emotion may feel too unsafe to stay with for more than a few seconds. They may wish to avoid going deeper or staying with their experiencing for very long. The humanistic sandtray therapist should not push or force the client to stay with emotions or go deeper if the client is showing signs of resistance. I discuss resistance later in this chapter. In HST, therapists value resistance because it can serve a protective function for a client.

Other clients may be cognitively oriented in such a way that entering emotions is a big step and staying with emotions is totally foreign. They may prefer to analyze an emotion. According to Armstrong (2008), "[c]lients cannot analyze a feeling and experience it at the same time" (p. 83). For example, a client who has built a scene symbolizing the death of a loved one may begin to feel sad, but then state, "I don't know why I can't just get over her death." Some therapists might respond with, "Tell me about that." However, that allows the client to stay in an analytical mode, which is the opposite aim of HST. Instead, to stay with the client's sadness and out of their head, I might use an exploratory question: "What is it like for you to grieve right now?"

For yet other clients, staying with may last a minute or more. The goal during these moments of intense emotional presence is to allow the client room to remain aware. Although seeking catharsis may be tempting for the therapist, that is not the goal. Therapeutic silence, presence, and eye contact are valuable skills as the client stays with and discovers.

Going Deeper into Emotion

When I teach graduate students and train therapists in HST, they often ask me, "How do I go deeper with a client?" It is a relevant question, no doubt. The process by which therapists co-navigate deeper into their clients' emotions is simple, but it can be challenging. However, there are some skills in HST that can be quite useful. As I have discussed, humanistic sandtray therapists design their responses with intention toward encouraging the client to *describe* or *notice* what comes up for them in the here and now (Armstrong, 2008). Examples of these kinds of therapist responses follow:

- As you think about that now, what do you notice?
- What is it like to feel such hurt right now?
- How are you distracting yourself right now?
- As you sit with your pain, what is coming up for you?
- Check out your anger. What do you notice?

Armstrong (2008) noted that going deeper into emotion allows clients to "experience feelings fully" (p. 81). He discussed some potential benefits to feeling fully. The first benefit is that feeling fully can help the client begin to accept and own their internal experiences rather than creating judgments about their emotions. Armstrong called this "being at home with myself" (p. 81). Another benefit is that it can help clients experience what a complete gestalt is like; in this case, completion of a gestalt of the figure—emotion arising, such as sadness, staying with sadness, and going deeper into sadness as it recedes into the ground. The more that humanistic sandtray therapists can assist clients experience an entire gestalt cycle, the less fearful they become of their emotions. Rogers (1989) echoed the importance of feeling an emotion fully and stated that once "a troubling feeling has been felt to its full depth and breadth, one can move on. It is an important part of movement in the process of change" (p. 151). Two additional strategies for going deeper into emotional experiencing are accentuating the obvious and body awareness.

Accentuating the Obvious

In *accentuating the obvious*, the humanistic sandtray therapist asks the client to exaggerate some feeling or movement to feel it more intensely (Armstrong, 2008). Because humanistic sandtray therapists trust in the paradoxical theory of change, they believe that directing clients to exaggerate their here-and-now experiencing provides clients with observations of how strongly they influence their own emotional state. There are three common ways in which humanistic sandtray therapists direct their clients to accentuate the obvious. One way is to ask the client to exaggerate their feeling (Armstrong, 2008). I might ask a client who feels sick when she begins talking about the miniature representing her boss to feel as disgusted as she possibly can. I might have her increase her disgust even more, a second time, while shifting her attention to *how* she is getting herself to feel such intensity.

Another way to direct clients to accentuate the obvious is to have them repeat something they just said that seems figural (Armstrong, 2008). Polster and Polster (1973) referred to this directed awareness as "accentuation of that which exists" (p. 225). This accentuation can be particularly therapeutic for clients who make statements that appear incongruent because they say something that seems meaningful to them but exhibit a neutral or mismatched emotion. Imagine a client tells her therapist that she feels grateful for the support her brother has provided during a period of her unemployment, and the therapist notices she said this as if she were reading a news report, in a factual manner. The therapist might ask her to say it again and experiment with saying it like she really means it. The point of this accentuation is to explore the client's emotional experience behind her statement because the therapist senses it has significance for the client.

Owning Experiences through Language

One of the benefits of going deeper into emotions with clients is that they begin to perceive how they influence their own experiencing. In HST, clinicians can help clients *own their experiences* by directing clients' attention to distancing language and suggesting alternatives that bring clients closer to self rather than their concepts (Armstrong, 2008). Many people tend to use second person when discussing their own experiences; for example, a client might say, "After mom died, you do what you have to do to get by." Clients use second person to avoid owning their own experiences because of the hurt involved with being close to their painful emotions. Humanistic sandtray therapists assist clients to own their experiences by gently asking them to experiment with using I-language instead of using second person: "After mom died, I did what I had to do to get by." Another way that clients use language to distance themselves is to remark on an experience as if it is in the past. A shift toward owning experiences can happen when you encourage clients to use the present tense: "After mom died, I'm doing what I have to do to get by." A third way that clients avoid owning their experiences is through using *must*, *have to*, and *can't*. These words symbolize shouldistic rather than organismic experiencing. In HST, therapists ask clients to experiment with changing this language that represents internal rules for restricting experiencing: "After mom died, I'm doing what I choose to get by." Another way of changing shouldistic language is to suggest that the client replaces *can't* with *won't* or *unwilling to*. It is important that you assist clients in being genuine and accurate with what they say because people tend to attach themselves strongly to the language that they use.

Enactment

Enactment is a form of accentuating the obvious that adds "dramatization within the therapy scene of some aspect of the patient's existence. It may start from a statement [they] make, or from a gesture" (Polster & Polster, 1973, pp. 239–240). Polster and Polster noted that enactment by nature is exhibitionistic. An important rationale behind enactment is that it allows the client to fully experience in the consultation room without an expectation that the client behaves in that manner outside of therapy.

For example, during a live demonstration of HST, one of my trainees included in her tray a small chimpanzee dressed in an astronaut uniform that she identified as herself. I asked her what it is like to monkey around. She said she feels foolish inside. If I had asked her to engage in enactment, I would have asked her to act as if she were the chimp in the space costume. I would have directed her to get up, be a chimpanzee and be a real fool, as foolish and as monkeyish as she could be in the moment. Some clients may respond with embarrassment or a sense of ridiculousness to enactment; however, exploring the limits of a client's emotion or concept can bring them to awareness of the performance aspect of their incongruent acts (Carson, 2003). In my trainee's case, her concept of herself as a dancing fool was utter bullshit stemming from her tendency to introject.

Body Awareness

In HST, one way of going deeper into emotional experiencing is to direct the client's awareness to their body. Armstrong (2008) stated that "*feelings are physical*" (p. 83; italics his). People are not always aware of feeling emotions in their bodies until they turn their attention toward these sensations. I learned this concept early on in my clinical training. When I was a graduate student in my second semester of clinical internship, my supervisor and I were watching a video recording I had with a client in which the client was tearful. My supervisor suggested to me that next time my client teared up, to say something along the lines of, "I see a tear forming in your eye. Take a moment and feel your tear fall down your cheek." At the time, the thought of saying that to a client felt too intimate to me. However, I gave it a shot, and the client was able to really experience her sadness and grief in that moment.

If a client expresses feeling anxious or worried, I might ask them, "Where in your body do you feel most worried right now?" I might also direct them to increase their bodily sense of anxiety, which is another way to accentuate the obvious in HST:

Client: In my hands. They are literally shaking right now when I hold them up.

Therapist: Try something. Hold your hands up. Allow them to shake without trying to change anything. What kind of sensations do you notice?

Client: My hands are suspended, and they have some kind of energy in them.

Therapist: So, right now you notice your hands are feeling unsupported yet ready for something. Why don't you shake them as much as you possibly can right now to see how ready you can make them?

Client: [*Shakes hands exaggeratingly*]

Therapist: What's it like to shake them like that?

Client: Actually, somehow, I feel like my hands are more prepared or something. I don't know. It's like my worry changed to excitement.

Therapist: You notice that you feel excited right now and you're not quite sure how you got there. Stay with your excitement for a moment.

In this example, the therapist engages in using reflection, exploratory questions, directed awareness, and accentuation of the obvious to bring the client into the guiding into–staying with–going deeper cycle. Some clients have easier access to their body, especially if they have introjected a self-limiting concept that "emotions are bad." In addition, some clients may notice how they are stopping themselves from feeling or "constricting the area in which they experience the feeling" (Armstrong, 2008, p. 84). For example, many clients restrict emotions like anger and sadness. If you ask a client who restricts anger to identify where in their bodies they experience anger, the client may report a sense of tightness not due to anger but due to their efforts to retroflect. Body awareness can lead to further discoveries of a client's *how* related to their emotional processing, polarities, and resistance.

Contraindicators of Going Deeper into Emotion

Some clients present with contraindicators of going deeper into emotion (Armstrong, 2008). Clients who are experiencing chronic and continuous trauma, such as people in active relationships characterized by intimate partner violence or other kinds of abusive relationships, are not appropriate for the kind of work I have been discussing. It is best to wait until they have exited those relationships and reach a level of emotional safety that allows them to tolerate feeling fully. In addition, some clients who have been diagnosed with personality disorders may be able to behaviorally demonstrate the responses that look like awareness and emotional experiencing; however, they may be quite detached from their actual internal experience due to a fragile or shattered ego. I advise caution in using these approaches with clients whom you assess as disconnected from reality.

Working within the Metaphor

A great strength of sandtray therapy is the opportunity to work within the metaphor of the tray (Armstrong, 2008; Homeyer & Sweeney, 2023). In HST, when *working within the metaphor*, therapists capitalize on the power of the here and now, facilitative and exploratory skills, and the guiding into–staying with–going deeper cycle of emotional experiencing. Unfortunately, metaphor work is also tempting for the therapist to interpret symbols. As I have discussed, our role is not to interpret. However, a good humanistic sandtray therapist does actively form and revise their *conceptualization* of the client's process in the tray. The sandtray scene is symbolic of the client's figure and ground. The totality of the scene initially forms ground and, alongside the creation and processing phases, what was ground becomes figural. Therefore, the scene, the miniatures, the sand, and the relational dynamics symbolized in the tray are intertwined in the client's figure–ground experience.

In HST, therapists approach metaphor work at multiple levels of depth in accordance with Bratton, Ceballos, and Webb Ferebee's (2009) system based on Oaklander's (2015) gestalt play therapy. Level one is the safest and entails asking the client to tell the therapist about their sandtray scene. In level two, the therapist offers their observations of the scene. You might comment on something the client mentioned or point out a figure or dynamic in the tray that the client has not discussed: "I see there is a fence surrounding the evil queen and she is looking directly at the house in which you dream of living." During level two metaphor work, it is important for the therapist to stay in the metaphor, commenting on miniatures in the ways that the client described them. If the client labels a miniature as their significant other, for example, that label is what you use. Similarly, when a client calls a miniature by its descriptor, such as "the fire engine," the therapist mirrors that language. Level three metaphor work entails inviting the client into the metaphor and, at times, experimenting with enactment. For example, sometimes when clients describe their scenes they do not identify where they are in the scene, whereupon I might say, "I wonder where you are in the scene." Also, I might say, "It seems like you feel trapped between your mother behind the fence and your aspirations inside your dream house." Finally, level four processing involves personalizing the metaphor and connecting it to the client's therapeutic themes: "I notice the figure who represents you is facing away from everyone else. What is it like for you to turn away?" Like other components of HST that seem stepwise, follow your client's lead. Some clients may describe their scenes from a level two or three point of view, so begin from that depth.

Polarities

Many theories of psychotherapy recognize that opposites lie at the core of human experience. From a gestalt perspective, people are "a never-ending sequence of polarities" (Polster & Polster, 1973, p. 61). Individuals develop unique systems of polarities that contribute to the formation of who they are and how they experience self and the situation. Often, people are aware of one side of a polarity but not the other side. For example, I recently started working with a dietitian to improve my eating and exercise habits, a recommendation from my primary care physician. When I first started, I was aware of my need to lose weight and ensure my overall physical health as I traipse toward my mid-forties. Related to my need to eat better was my competing need to eat enjoyable meals and snacks. I am several weeks into these new eating habits, and I feel a tight tension, even as I write this sentence, of my polarity: I want to take care of my body, *and* I want to have no boundaries around my eating. Related to this values-based polarity is an emotional polarity: I feel disappointed in my body, *and* I feel content in my body as-is. Notice that I used the word "and" to connect the two sides of each polarity. What many people tend to do is use the word "but" if they recognize both sides of their polarity at all. An issue with "but" is that it minimizes and devalues the first part of the polarity. *Both sides of a polarity have value* (Armstrong, 2008). There are many other kinds of polarities that people have within them. Examples are survivor-victim, fulfilled-overwhelmed, and well-behaved-naughty. Thematically, polarities tend to be related to "two opposing tendencies, parts, wants or desires" (Armstrong, 2008, p. 95), self-concept (Zinker, 1977), and I would add emotions and values. Polarities are idiosyncratic and most of the time, the other side of the polarity is implied—the side that the client does not want to recognize or of which they are afraid.

In HST, polarities arise not only when clients talk about themselves. They also symbolize them in their trays. Typically, the astute humanistic sandtray therapist can observe both sides of a client's polarity in their trays. I am having trouble thinking about a time when I did not observe a polarity in a client's tray. An almost sure sign of a polarity is when clients use bridges, fences, walls, or a line of gems or rocks. Another way clients symbolize polarities is through positioning of miniatures in the tray. Miniatures that face away from each other or miniatures that are visually or characteristically opposite in nature, such as fire and water or an evil character and a good character, are also typical ways to capture polarities. In addition, clients may include clusters of objects representing polarities (Armstrong, 2008). There may be a group of miniatures about the past and another about the present or future, or there may be a scene within the scene of joy and one of sadness.

Furthermore, polarities may emerge when going deeper into emotional experiencing. A client may notice feeling sad and yet also tighten their throat to stop from crying. They feel sad but also feel afraid to cry. Here, I purposefully used the word "but" to describe the client's midst of an active polarity. This kind of polarity is related to resistance, which I will discuss later in this chapter. Another example comes from my experience working with clients who are grieving, especially when the nature of their relationship with their loved one was defined by polarities. For example, imagine that in her tray a client depicted a polarity that a part of her felt sad and another part of her felt relief that her husband was dead. These two emotions are in conflict. The client's late husband was emotionally abusive for many years and there was plenty of meaning in her feelings of relief, but she is afraid to acknowledge them because she believes she *should only feel sadness* due to her introjection of society's expectations, and to feel relief would mean she is a bad person. A client like this is likely to report an inability to fully feel the part of her that feels sad. Clients often have concepts about the "right" way to feel, and this leads to a shouldistic way of functioning, causing rigidity in their living.

When humanistic sandtray therapists work with polarities, ultimately their therapeutic goal is to integrate both parts (Armstrong, 2008). However, before integrating two opposing parts, the therapist must work with the client to identity their polarity, separate the parts, and accept both parts. Polster and Polster (1973) stated that "[t]he task in resolving the polarity is to aid each part to live to its fullest while at the same time making contact with its polar counterpart" (p. 63). However, because clients are often afraid to acknowledge the part that they tend to minimize or downplay, polarities work can be challenging. Integrating a polarity takes time and energy and may take months. I now move to discussing each of four steps in polarities work as proposed by Armstrong (2008).

Identifying, Naming, and Acknowledging the Polarity

The first step in polarities work is to help the client observe, name, and acknowledge the polarity. Returning to the example of the bereaved female client whose emotionally abusive husband died, her stuckness with grief is related to her polarity. Initial identification of her polarity may arise from my observations or hers. She and I would work together to name her polarity. Naming of a polarity is patterned typically as

I want/feel/need _____, but I can't/I'm afraid to/I don't want to/it's hard to _____.

After naming the polarity, I would then check with the client to ensure its accuracy. If the client states that the polarity fits with her conceptually, then I would move on to step two. If the client states that it does not quite fit, I would encourage her to rename it, or we might continue exploring to find a better name. Following is an example of how step one might go.

Client: [*While describing her tray*] Right here in the corner, the faceless person, is me.

Therapist: So, there's no expression on your face there. What is that like?

Client: It's sad. That person there really is sad. There is more to me though. That's why there's this stuff in the other corner, where the line of trees is. Behind it is a little pool of water, like a little relaxing place just for me. But it's hidden.

Therapist: Okay, and you as the faceless person are staring right at that line of trees. It seems like part of you is feeling sad about your late husband's death and part of you is feeling or wants to feel ... relaxed?

Client: Yes, but I shouldn't be wanting to relax right now. I mean, Ron just died two months ago.

Therapist: What I'm hearing is that part of you feels sad, and part of you feels relieved, too. Is that right?

Client: Yeah, but I don't think I should be feeling that way. Isn't it a terrible thing to feel relieved that someone is dead? Especially the person I spent 24 years with?

Therapist: I see. You want to feel relieved, but you're afraid that if you do it means you're a bad person.

Client: That's exactly it.

Therapist: Okay. Say that out loud and let me know what comes up for you. "I want to feel relief, but I'm afraid that if I do it means I'm a bad person."

Client: I want to feel relief, but I'm afraid that if I do it means I'm bad.

Therapist: [*Silence*] How are you reacting to that?

Client: Yes, and I get so stuck in it. I'm stuck in it now.

In the example above, it took a little bit of exploration between me and the client to settle on the polarity. This is an example with a relatively self-aware client. However, clients who lack self-awareness can be challenging even in step one because they may not even be aware that the opposing part lies within them. They may be more likely to externalize or assign responsibility to others for the opposing part. Other times, as the therapist, I may have difficulty capturing what the client is communicating with each side of the polarity and therefore misname it. It is important to stay present and patient during polarities work. If the polarity is an important force in the client's life, there will be additional opportunities to explore and name it.

Separating and Exploring the Parts

Once the client finds a good fit with the name of a polarity and acknowledges its presence within them, then the therapist moves to step two, separating and exploring the parts. Polster and Polster (1973) suggested that a two-chair or an empty chair dialogue is a typical experiment to use in separation and exploration. Armstrong (2008) noted that empty chair could be useful with adults during sandtray work. In my experience, a two-chair dialogue can be especially useful in sandtray because the therapist can direct action to the parts of the tray that symbolize the client's polarity, even without having a physical chair in the room! However, I caution you that it is best practice to receive focused training in two-chair and empty chair dialogue before using them with clients. These experiments are beyond the scope of this book because of their danger if used improperly.

Another way of separating and exploring parts is to *assess the presence of opposing parts* within the client's here-and-now experiencing. Returning to the bereaved client and her polarity, an example of assessing the presence follows.

Therapist: Right now, you're feeling stuck between the part of you that feels relief and the part of you that is afraid to feel this fully. Which are you more aware of right now, the part of you that feels relief or the part of you that feels afraid?

Client: Oh, definitely the part that feels afraid.

Therapist: Describe what you're experiencing with your fear right now.

Client: It's like I'm on the edge of a cliff looking over. If I step off, then I'll never come back.

Therapist: Where do you feel your edge of a cliff fear in your body?

Client: Here, in the pit of my stomach.

Therapist: I wonder if you'd try something. Place your hand on your stomach, right where the pit of fear is. See if you can press your hand into that pit, so that you can almost touch it.

When the therapist assesses the presence of opposing parts, they are inviting the client to experience their emerging figure. The therapist then has many options for exploration with an emphasis on the guiding into–staying with–going deeper cycle. Typically, once a client has experienced one part, the other part tends to emerge, and the therapist guides the client into exploration.

Accepting Both Parts

Typically, therapist and client will only engage in the first two steps of the polarities process during the sandtray session. Step three takes time and effort and will likely become one of the thematic focuses of further therapy sessions. Accepting both parts of a polarity takes a lot of courage, focused energy, and awareness on the part of the client and therapist. According to Armstrong (2008):

Acceptance of different parts of ourselves can be quite difficult and take a long time even if we are willing to own both parts. I say if we are willing to own both parts because many people are not willing to do this. Many people are tremendously ashamed of parts of themselves ... We tend to hide parts of which we are ashamed.

(p. 102)

In addition, as clients are working to accept both parts, they may behave in unexpected ways because they can become confused about which part is really them as well as how to act (Polster & Polster, 1973). Clients may become resistant or defensive out of fear of accepting all parts of themselves and learning how to experience and behave based on a continuum rather than a singular rigid standard or concept. When people find themselves facing all parts of themselves, especially the parts they despise or feel guilty or shame about, they often recoil and go back to older patterns of conceiving themselves and behaving. Sometimes familiarity is safer than the unknown, particularly when the unknown is within self. Therefore, accepting both parts can be a trying, risky, and unpleasant phase of humanistic therapy. My hope when working with clients with acceptance is that they will find significantly more contentment with self and environment as they work toward the final step, integrating the parts.

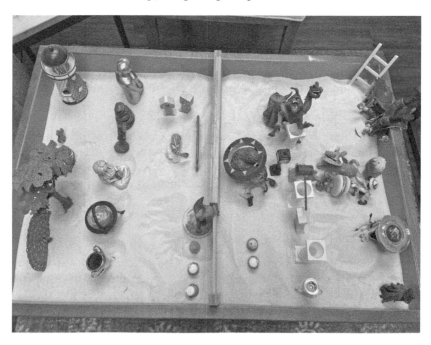

Figure 4.1 Client's sandtray as they work to accept both parts of their polarity.

Integrating the Parts

Clients have a long way to go and a lot of therapeutic work to do as they integrate their parts (Armstrong, 2008). Not all my clients make it this far. Some terminate therapy before they get here, or they resolve some major issues, yet their deep-seated polarities remain. When clients make it to this step of polarities work, they have stopped most denial mechanisms, accepted that they have conflicting parts, and faced both experientially while remaining courageous and open. Depending on where a client began in their journey toward awareness, it may only take a few months to integrate their parts. Others may take longer. Integration, like accepting both parts, requires steadfast attunement to a deep therapeutic relationship and application of the guiding into–staying with–going deeper cycle. What therapists will witness with their clients is that they begin to become less fearful about exploration of self and experience a surge in stamina and creativity in their awareness process.

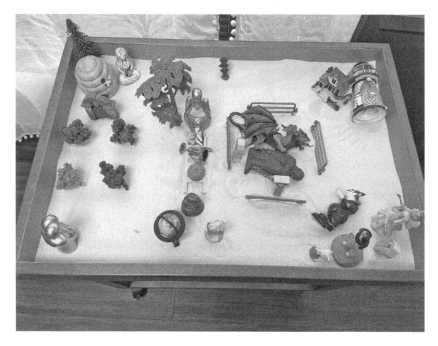

Figure 4.2 Client's sandtray as they begin to integrate both parts of their polarity.

Resistance

The topic of resistance has shown up in the psychotherapy literature since Freud. It is not an alien concept to most therapists, and I would bet that running into client resistance can be one of the more frustrating aspects of clinical practice. Sometimes, therapists create their own feelings of irritation or stuckness when they encounter resistance because they have their clients' best interests in mind and deeply care about their client changing in order to feel better. Most therapists have no desire to see their clients struggle or remain stagnant. Some therapists discuss client resistance as a negative characteristic. I have even heard therapists talk about clients in pejorative and blaming ways when clients resist. Yet other therapists invest too much of their self-concept and self-efficacy into client outcome.

The humanistic view of resistance is that it is there for a meaningful reason. Resistance can have a positive function in a client's life (Mann, 2021; Polster & Polster, 1973) by protecting them from toxic environments. However, as with all parts of human functioning, resistance can also become dysfunctional, particularly in relationships with people who are relatively healthy. And, of course, resistance can be an obstacle in the therapeutic relationship. Armstrong (2008) noted that "[r]esistance is almost always an outward manifestation of a polarity in the client: *the client wants to change and is afraid to change*" (p. 110; italics his). From this point of view, resistance is rooted in fear and, therefore, in a psychotherapy situation emerges as figural when clients feel anxious or perceptually threatened emotionally. Resistance is incredibly typical in psychotherapy and is an integral part of humanistic work. I can say with a fair degree of accuracy that every client I have worked with has demonstrated resistance at some point during our work together. When I feel myself getting frustrated in my work with a client and invest energy into reflection, I often discover client resistance. Then, I introduce patience and grace into the therapeutic relationship and shift back into an exploration mode with the client.

In HST, the basic approach to resistance is to *allow the client to have their defenses*. Armstrong (2008) framed this approach as going "*with the resistance rather than against it*" (p. 109; italics his). Because polarities underlie resistance, the HST approach is to follow the four-step polarities process outlined earlier in this chapter. Allow me to provide an example.

Imagine that I am working with a Latina cisgendered heterosexual client in her thirties. She initially presented with symptoms of depression and anxiety related to her marriage. Several sessions in, she begins to think about the possibility of separating from her husband because of his history of having multiple affairs and his verbally abusive behavior toward my client. I invite her to create a sandtray scene and I notice two opposing parts: a fire-breathing dragon representing her husband and a fearful looking miniature representing herself. As she discusses the scene, I sense a feeling of "YES!" in my body, but I do my best to maintain a neutral position. I feel tempted to encourage her to leave and begin offering resources to her.

In this instance, I am reacting how I imagine other therapists might react when they sense their client is on the edge of making decisions that, in the therapist's opinion, are good.

However, going down a pathway of helping my client get out of her situation withdraws her autonomy and totally overlooks the potential significance of her own defenses. She has not left him yet, after many years of behaviors with which she disagrees fervently and by which she feels deeply hurt. Why has she not left him yet? Beyond the many practical reasons, her intrapersonal reason likely has to do with *fear*. Therefore, following step one in the polarities process, I work with my client to identify, name, and acknowledge her polarity: "I want to leave my husband, but I'm afraid to."

Moving into step two of the polarities process, I would work with her to separate and explore each part. She is probably well aware of her desire to leave her husband as she has been discussing her wish for the last several sessions and has placed it in the tray. Once she acknowledges her polarity, I would assess the presence of her opposing parts by asking her which part she is most aware of in the moment. At some point her fear will be figural for her, and I would invite her into directed awareness to accentuate that which exists, her fear of leaving. We would explore that side of her polarity. Often clients in this kind of situation might say something like, "I can't leave because _____ (I can't afford financially to live on my own; I don't want our kids to suffer)." I would have her repeat her statement about her perceived inability to leave. Here, I am opening a space for my client to feel her fear fully. I might notice that my client is tiptoeing into her fear by stopping her experience. I would likely guide her into body awareness and accentuate the way she is stopping herself from fully feeling her fear and anxiety. Another option would be to ask her, "How are you stopping yourself from feeling fearful right now?"

There are multiple ways to engage in polarities work to address resistance within the four-step model; as long as the therapist allows the client to have their experience, even if their experience is defensiveness or guardedness, then the process is unfolding according to humanistic principles. The worst move here is to try to make the client do or experience something that they feel unsafe to face in the moment. Remember that change is paradoxical. Clients are more likely to change when they feel a sense of freedom within the therapeutic relationship rather than a sense of force from the therapist. Clients should on themselves enough without the therapist's help. This idea may sound like I am suggesting that therapists allow clients to escape responsibility. On the contrary, the HST process is heavily invested in bringing clients *at choice* where they are aware of their responsibility to respond in a new way—or not—and akin to the concept of returning responsibility in child-centered play therapy (Landreth, 2023).

Conclusion

Armstrong (2008) stated that "[w]orking with feelings on a deep level is difficult. It is difficult for clients and difficult for therapists because this kind of work can be somewhat unpredictable" (p. 82). Although I have reviewed multiple steps and processes that I use in HST, because my main goal is exploration and discovery, it is nearly impossible for me to know ahead of time how a client will respond or what new material and experiencing will surface. The facilitation, reflection, and directed awareness skills and strategies I outlined in this chapter can be powerful and lead a client into vulnerable places that they have yet to fully experience, requiring great sensitivity, compassion, attunement, presence, and patience from the humanistic sandtray therapist. The mechanics of the HST approach take focused, reflective practice and have potential to contribute to meaningful client change.

References

Armstrong, S. A. (2008). *Sandtray therapy: A humanistic approach*. Ludic Press.

Beisser, A. (1970). The paradoxical theory of change. In J. Fagan & I. L. Shepherd (Eds.), *Gestalt therapy now: Theories, techniques, applications* (pp. 77–80). Science and Behavior Books.

Bratton, S. C., Ceballos, P. L., & Webb Ferebee, K. (2009). Integration of structured expressive activities within a humanistic group play therapy format for preadolescents. *The Journal for Specialists in Group Work, 34*(3), 251–275. https://doi.org/10.1080/01933920903033487

Carson, R. (2003). *Taming your gremlin: A surprisingly simple method for getting out of your own way* (Revised ed.). William Morrow.

Landreth, G. L. (2023). *Play therapy: The art of the relationship* (4th ed.). Routledge. https://doi.org/10.4324/9781003255796

Mann, D. (2021). *Gestalt therapy: 100 key points and techniques* (2nd ed.). Routledge. https://doi.org/10.4324/9781315158495

Oaklander, V. (2015). *Windows to our children* (35th anniversary ed.). The Gestalt Journal Press.

Polster, E., & Polster, M. (1973). *Gestalt therapy integrated: Contours of theory & practice*. Brunner/Mazel.

Rogers, C. R. (1989). A client-centered/person-centered approach to therapy. In H. Kirschenbaum & V. L. Henderson (Eds.), *The Carl Rogers reader* (pp. 135–156). Houghton Mifflin.

Stevens, C. (2004). Playing in the sand. *The British Gestalt Journal, 13*(1), 18–23.

Zinker, J. (1977). *Creative process in Gestalt therapy*. Brunner/Mazel.

Chapter 5

Neurobiology, Trauma, and Humanistic Sandtray Therapy

Ryan D. Foster and L. Marinn Pierce

> Nervous systems came late in the history of life. No, nervous systems were not primary on any count. Nervous systems showed up to serve life, to make life possible, when the complexity of organisms required high levels of functional coordination. And yes, nervous systems helped generate remarkable phenomena and functions that were not present before their arrival such as feelings, minds, consciousness, explicit reasoning, verbal languages, and mathematics.
>
> —Damasio, 2021, p. 23

Beginning in the third week of gestation, the human brain starts to develop as cells divide and differentiate into neurons and glia, forming the foundation of the nervous system. Although the foundation of human brain development occurs in utero, this development will continue into early adulthood with the periods of greatest development occurring from conception to age two and late adolescence to early adulthood. Brain development after birth occurs primarily through relational and sensory input. These periods of development are followed by a period of synaptic pruning during which time the brain organizes and reduces synaptic connections to increase efficiency and productivity (Konkel, 2018; Perry & Szalavitz, 2006). Brain development is influenced by intersections of genetics and environment—social, physical, relational, and environmental—and evidence demonstrates that psychotherapy can influence this development over the lifespan (Badenoch, 2008). Moreover, contemporary psychotherapists from a variety of theoretical approaches have theorized that sand therapies can have a powerful impact on neurobiological structures and mechanisms because they are holistic approaches involving emotion, thinking, and sensorimotor capacities, which involve several major areas of the human brain (Dawson, 2024; Fraser, 2022; Gonzalo Marrodán & Moraga, 2024; Grayson, 2022). In particular, sand therapists frequently frame sand therapy practice as an effective method for helping clients heal trauma because sand therapies can have a profound impact on attachment mechanisms (Badenoch, 2008).

DOI: 10.4324/9781032664996-6

Humanistic sandtray therapy (HST) is an approach that is well-suited for clients whose neurobiological systems have been impacted by trauma. In this chapter, we will provide a rationale for the use of HST with clients who have experienced trauma based on a conceptual understanding of neurophysiology, polyvagal theory, interpersonal neurobiology, and attachment. We will also provide a rationale establishing HST as a trauma-informed approach to mental health care.

Neurophysiology

The nervous system is composed of more than 100 billion neurons and trillions of support cells called glia. Because every neuron can have up to 10,000 connections, it is estimated that the nervous system consists of over a quadrillion connections (Edelman & Tononi, 2000). The nervous system includes two subsystems: the central nervous system (CNS) and the peripheral nervous system (PNS; Heller & LaPierre, 2012; Perry & Szalavitz, 2006). The CNS consists of the brain and spinal cord whereas the PNS includes the nerves and ganglia existing beyond the spinal cord and brain. Although researchers offer these dictions for conceptualization, the CNS and PNS are highly dependent on one another and function as a unit.

The Central Nervous System

In the 1960s, the model of the triune brain was developed by Paul MacLean (1990), who proposed that the human brain actually contained three different "brains." Now considered an oversimplified understanding, it still can be helpful for conceptualization. Based on this model, the brain is divided into three distinct sections: the reptilian brain, the paleomammalian brain or limbic system, and the neocortex (Shanker, 2016). The brainstem sits at the base of the brain and connects the brain to the spinal cord (Miller-Karas, 2015). In fact, some professionals consider the brainstem to be part of the spinal cord (Habib, 2019). The brainstem develops in utero and is responsible for regulating autonomic functions, such as heartbeat, respiration, pain sensitivity, and alertness (Heller & LaPierre, 2012). Additionally, all information communicated between the body and the brain travels through the brainstem. This function allows the brainstem to have a critical role in survival, as it has the capacity to enter into defensive responses when the body is under perceived threat, without engaging the slower, more complex areas of the brain. The thalamus is just above the brainstem. It relays sensory information connected to taste, sight, touch, and hearing to the appropriate parts of the brain. The cerebellum, at the back of the brainstem, processes non-verbal implicit memory and is responsible for the coordination of voluntary movement (Miller-Karas, 2015). The basal ganglia supports procedural memory (Heller & LaPierre, 2012). It should be noted that one or all of these parts of the brain are referred to as the reptilian brain, depending on the perspective of the speaker.

The limbic system developed with the evolution of mammals and surrounds the brainstem (Heller & LaPierre, 2012). This system has critical functions in relationships, emotion, and memory and includes the amygdala, hippocampus, hypothalamus, and the striatum (Shanker, 2016). The amygdala is responsible for processing emotions such as fear and anxiety. If a situation is perceived as dangerous, the amygdala has the capacity to initiate a danger signal without conscious awareness, thus activating a stress response (Miller-Karas, 2015). The hippocampus functions in the storage and organization of explicit memory and moving memories from short-term to long-term (Doidge, 2007). The hypothalamus regulates the autonomic nervous system and is responsible for the secretion of hormones through the endocrine system (Miller-Karas, 2015). Part of the hypothalamic-pituitary-adrenal (HPA) axis, the hypothalamus connects the brain to the endocrine system through the pituitary gland, which sits just below it. The adrenal glands, each of which sits on top of a kidney, are responsible for firing stress hormones (Heller & LaPierre, 2012). The striatum is responsible for processing movement (Doidge, 2007).

Lastly, the neocortex consists of the most complex parts of the brain and contains four lobes: the frontal lobe, the parietal lobe, the occipital lobe, and the temporal lobe. The occipital, parietal, and temporal lobes are responsible for processing sensory information. The occipital and temporal lobes process visual and auditory information, respectively, whereas the parietal lobe processes sensory information related to touch and body movements. The frontal lobe contains multiple parts and is responsible for rational thinking, problem-solving, and future planning. This function includes the motor strip, which controls the planning and completion of motor function. The motor strip works closely with the premotor, which is responsible for spatial awareness, in controlling motor movements (Miller-Karas, 2015). The anterior circulate cortex (ACC) and insula have functions in the processing of empathy and the ability to focus attention (Doidge, 2007). The insula, in particular, supports the function of interoception. Lastly, the prefrontal cortex and orbital-frontal cortex are responsible for the organization of thoughts, strategizing, and moral decision-making. A more developed neocortex has the potential to regulate the function of the limbic system (Miller-Karas, 2015).

HST and the CNS

HST has the potential to activate major areas of the CNS. When a client constructs a tray by manipulating the miniatures, touching the sand,

and seeing their three-dimensional scene, these sensory inputs are directed through the thalamus and the occipital, temporal, and parietal lobes. An adult client with a developed neocortex may find that their sensory experiences during the creation phase of HST can activate an anxiety response in their amygdala as they observe sandtray scenes that represent vulnerable experiences. However, during the processing phase, through increased awareness that opens clients to observing their scenes from a new experiential point of view, these same sensory systems in the neocortex may also assist in regulating the amygdala during fear states.

The Peripheral Nervous System

The PNS is composed of two divisions. The afferent sensory division relays information from the body to the PNS whereas the efferent motor division relays information from the PNS to the body. Within the efferent motor division exist two subsystems – the somatic motor system (SMS), which is responsible for the voluntary movements of our muscles, and the autonomic nervous system (ANS; Heller & LaPierre, 2012). From a psychotherapeutic perspective, the ANS appears to have a particularly intriguing role in the work that we do with clients.

From the earliest moments of gestation, the ANS is developing. The ANS is responsible for the regulation of involuntary, physiological functions and relays messages from the central nervous system to the organs and glands of the body. Focused in the brainstem and vagus nerve, the ANS is responsible for respiration, heart rate, digestion, sleep, and arousal, including sexual arousal (Waxenbaum, Reddy, & Varacallo, 2023). It helps regulate the activation and rest functions. The arousal function supports the body in response to threats. As such, the ANS is impacted often by trauma, particularly with regard to how these brain functions influence a client's subsequent interactions in relationships (Kain & Terrell, 2018).

The Traditional View of the ANS

Within the traditional view of the autonomic nervous system, there are two primary subsystems: the sympathetic nervous system and the parasympathetic nervous system. There is an additional third system, the enteric nervous system, which can function independently and is responsible for digestive functions. The sympathetic nervous system and parasympathetic nervous system relay incoming sensory information and outgoing motor movements to and from the CNS (Waxenbaum et al., 2023). When activated, the sympathetic nervous system initiates the "fight or flight" response and is present in almost every part of the human body. During this process, glycogenolysis, a process of metabolizing stored glycogen in the liver for energic use, is initiated. Heart rate, blood pressure, and respiration increase in order to transport this energy to the necessary parts of the body. All other functions deemed non-essential for threat survival cease, including digestion. The parasympathetic nervous system, however, is much smaller and is present in the head, viscera, and external genitals. Responsible for what is commonly referred to as "rest and digest," the parasympathetic nervous system essentially serves the opposite function of the sympathetic nervous system in lowering the heart rate, blood pressure, and respiration, and activating digestion and other non-essential functions.

The responses of the ANS exist along a continuum from deep rest to a flooded fight response. Throughout the day, humans fluctuate along this continuum. Ideally, theses transitions are smooth with the vast majority of time spent within the middle of the continuum and creating minimal disruption in daily life; however, at times, a system can become hyper-fixated in a state, thus, taxing the system (Shanker, 2016)—a common result of trauma. From this perspective, arousal can be measured through blood pressure, heart rate, or respiration and this arousal is connected to activity in the limbic and cortical areas of the brain; therefore, assumptions can be made about the limbic system and neocortex through the measurement of autonomic responses (Porges, 2021).

Polyvagal Theory

Porges (2011) challenged the traditional view of the ANS. Porges (2021) stated that:

> Polyvagal Theory was introduced as an attempt to shift the science of psychophysiology from a descriptive science conducting empirical studies and describing correlations between psychological and physiological processes to an inferential science generating and testing hypotheses related to common neural pathways involving both mental and physiological processes.
>
> (p. 2)

He found the dualistic focus on only measurable data, like heart rate and blood pressure, to be limiting and posited that as vertebrates evolved so, too, did their mechanisms for survival. Thus, the focus of polyvagal theory is the phylogenetic modifications that developed as humans evolved from reptiles.

Porges (2011) hypothesized that the ANS is subdivided into three primary systems rather than two, as described by the traditional view. This additional subsystem is connected to mylenated versus unmyelnated portions of the vagus nerve. The vagus nerve begins in the brainstem and runs the length of the torso with branches connecting to areas of the auditory, respiratory, cardiovascular, and digestive systems. Approximately 80 percent of the function of the vagus is afferent, communicating information from the body to the brain (Habib, 2019). According to polyvagal theory, humans adapted three responses to threat. The first, and most primitive, is immobilization in which the individual feigns death. This response, often called the dorsal vagal response, is shared with most other vertebrates. Humans enter into a shutdown strategy that includes weakened muscle tone and lowered heart and respiration rates. According to Porges (2011), this response relies on the oldest branch of the vagus nerve, known as the dorsal motor nuecleus of the vagus, an unmylenated branch starting in the brainstem. Second is the sympathetic response described previously. Porges noted this response requires a "functioning" (p. 16) sympathetic nervous system. The third system, often referred to as the ventral vagus system, includes aspects of social engagement such as facial expressions and vocalization. Porges suggested this system was operated by a myelinated portion of the vagus originating in the nucleus ambigus area of the brainstem. From the perspective of survival, the purpose of the ventral vagus is to inhibit the sympathetic nervous system and settle the ANS.

Neuroception is the term coined by Porges (2011) to describe the process by which humans assess for safety and danger. This unconscious process takes place in the most primitive parts of the brain; therefore, before an individual has consciously assessed the level of threat, an adaptive sequence for survival already may be activated—either sympathetic activation or a dorsal vagal response of shutdown. Porges posited that systems assess the biological movements of others as well as auditory input, with particular emphasis on vocal prosody. Even light changes in a person or external or internal environment can shift the neuroception from safety to danger. In order to engage in prosocial behavior, the defensive strategies must be inhibited without immobilization. Therefore, social engagement, or ventral vagal, is a parasympathetic response of safety that requires inhibition of the defensive strategies of the sympathetic response while allowing for activation of the prosocial aspects of the sympathetic nervous system. Porges (2011) hypothesized that the prefrontal cortex and temporal cortex work closely with the amygdala to support neuroception. Faulty neuroception occurs when there is "an inaccurate assessment of the safety or danger of a situation" (Porges, 2011, p. 13).

HST and the ANS

Polyvagal theory acts as a conceptual lens through which humanistic sandtray therapists can understand how HST impacts a client's ability to influence their ANS through increased awareness and here-and-now experiencing.

Early in psychotherapeutic work, clients neuroceptively perceive a threat to safety as they create sandtray scenes that bring their background of experiencing to foreground. For clients who have well-established patterns of defense and resistance, their sympathetic nervous system response activates as early as the creation phase and most certainly during the processing phase as their heart rate increases, breathing shortens, and feelings of fear arise. During this activation, it is absolutely incumbent on the humanistic sandtray therapist to engage in deep empathic attunement and focus on exploration and discovery. Temporarily exiting the tray and entering into the felt sense with the client allows them to get to know *how* they are perceiving their vulnerability—likely as a threat and something that demands that they press their foot on the brakes of their experiencing. In the longer term, what humanistic sandtray therapists are attempting to do is invite clients into an opportunity to shift into ventral vagal and, thus, safety.

Explicit and Implicit Memory

Memory is the process of bringing the past to the present. The primary purpose of memory is to help the system assess for threat and respond as needed. Explicit memories are those that require intentional learning or retention of information and are processed primarily in the hippocampus and frontal lobes (Miller-Karas, 2015). Levine (2015) identified explicit memory to be either declarative or episodic. Declarative memories include factual, or relatively factual information, that is intentionally retained, and are the easiest memories to consciously call up. They often have little significant emotional connection. Examples include learned data and facts, historical stories, and even potentially the to-do list of the day. Episodic memories are those with emotional connections, both pleasant and unpleasant. Levine described these as more autobiographical and less conscious than declarative memories. They can be vague or vivid and more nuanced than declarative memories. Episodic memories help us orient to person, place, time, and space.

Implicit memories are unconscious memories that cannot be simply recalled. Like explicit memories, there are two types of implicit memories: emotional and procedural. Implicit memories serve the purpose of being stored for quick recall for safety and survival and are processed in the cerebellum and basal ganglia (Levine, 2015; Miller-Karas, 2015). Levine described these memories as powerful. Emotional memories serve as alerts or flags, filed away for recall to initiate a procedural response. There are three types of procedural memory: learned motor actions, emergency responses, and approach or avoidance. Learned motor actions are those behaviors that do not require higher order thinking to complete, like walking or chewing food. Emergency responses are fixed action patterns of constriction, fighting, fleeing, freezing, or immobilization. Lastly, approach or avoidance behaviors include those indicating impulse to retract from or move toward a person or situation. Procedural memory includes survival patterns and responses and can be conceptualized as conditioned or patterned responses. Implicit memories begin forming in the earliest moments of life.

HST and Memory Activation

Although in HST clients are encouraged to create trays that represent the present, inevitably there will be experiences and events that represent episodic and implicit memories. These memories are very much present for clients, however, in their minds, bodies, and sandtrays. How clients respond to their emotions, for example, is partially encoded in procedural memory, becoming a habitual part of a client's functioning. From a neurobiological point of view, clients' memories were encoded in the past, yet clients experience them in the here and now.

Interpersonal Neurobiology and Co-regulation

According to Shankar (2016), "[c]ompared with the rest of the animal kingdom, the human brain is remarkably immature for a remarkably long time" (p. 50). As noted previously, the most primitive functions of the nervous system develop in utero. The more complex, nuanced parts of the nervous system develop primarily during the first three years of life but will continue for decades following. In infancy, the only defensive strategy available to the system is that of immobilization. Infants initiate cries of distress related to necessities for daily functioning like food, sleep, or diaper change. Ideally, these cries are soothed through contact with a regulated, nurturing, attentive caregiver. The young system is soothed through gentle touch, rhythmic movements like rocking, and vocalization, particularly with prosody, offered in connection with another. This process is called co-regulation. If, however, the infant's cries are not responded to or the caregiver is misattuned, the stress response may not settle. As the infant is unable to complete a fight or flight response, likely they will shift into an immobilized response of shut down, which can appear as settled but is a very different nervous system response. As such, the process of learning self-regulation requires regular experiences of co-regulation. Humans continue to require capacities for co-regulation and self-regulation throughout the lifespan (Kain & Terrell, 2018; Perry & Szalavitz, 2006; Shankar, 2016).

Additionally, as infants experience these moments of attunement, oxytocin is released in the system. The secretion of this hormone during moments of nurture and engagement connects these experiences with moments of pleasure (Kain & Terrell, 2018). Porges (2011) hypothesized it is this procedural process that supports the social engagement of the ventral vagal process that allows humans later in life to experience immobilization of embrace, like cuddling or hugs, as safe rather than activating a threat response.

Neuroplasticity and Neurogenesis

Neuroplasticity is defined as the capacity of the brain to change or modify. Although this process can be complex and nuanced, two functions stand out: pruning and neurogenesis. Pruning is the process by which the brain removes those synaptic connections that are no longer necessary and allows for more efficient processing. Neurogenesis is the process of developing new synaptic connections (Miller-Karas, 2015). In 1949, Hebb theorized that neurons that fire simultaneously repeatedly will strengthen their synaptic connection. This theory is commonly referred to as the "fire together wire together" principle. Doidge (2007) reported significant differences in the motor cortex and the cerebellum between musicians and non-musicians, a larger hippocampus in London taxi drivers compared with the general population, and thicker insulas in meditators. Merzenich et al. (1999) found practicing a new skill impacted as many as hundreds of millions of connections.

HST, Neurobiology, and Co-regulation

Because HST emphasizes humanistic processes such as empathic attunement, warmth, authenticity, and presence, humanistic sandtray therapists in effect become experiential co-regulators to all clients when regulation systems experience too little or too much activation. This important role of humanistic sandtray therapists is one reason for such a strong focus on the processing phase of HST. The creation phase may activate these regulation systems, and without entering into the processing phase, clients whose neurobiological systems have no or limited pathways for self-regulation may be left vulnerable and activated without ventral vagal resolution. We suggest that compassionate exploration, here-and-now presence, and a focus on awareness during the processing phase of HST allow clients to experience co-regulation, thereby creating a new neurobiological model of self-regulation via neurogenesis.

Trauma and HST

Trauma-informed approaches to psychotherapy have proliferated in the professional literature over the last two decades. Perry and Szalavitz (2006) noted that "[e]xperience can become biology" (p. 1) and this is especially relevant for clients who have experienced one or more traumatic events. Steele and Malchiodi (2012) identified sandtray therapy as a trauma-informed approach because of its ability to activate attachment systems that are vulnerable to harmful impacts of trauma. Homeyer and Lyles (2022) outlined a number of recommendations for trauma work in the sand. Gonzalo Marrodán and Moraga (2024) outlined extensively their sandtray-trauma model. Although reviewing a complete history and rationale for trauma-informed approaches is beyond the scope of this book, our goal here is to give you guidance on how to apply HST with your clients who have experienced trauma. We will offer practical suggestions on how to adapt your sandtray materials and provide an inclusive environment for differences in sensory systems.

We frame our discussion using the Substance Abuse and Mental Health Services Administration's (SAMHSA, 2014) six principles for trauma-informed approaches: safety; trustworthiness and transparency; peer support; collaboration and mutuality; empowerment, voice, and choice; and cultural, historical, and gender issues. SAMHSA developed these six principles as a result of decades of research demonstrating that trauma is widespread among those with mental health concerns and impacts not only their daily functioning but their ability to access quality mental health care. SAMHSA intends its trauma-informed approach to transcend mental health care systems by encouraging public institutions across the service spectrum to employ their guidance. Likewise, we believe that HST is inherently a trauma-informed approach and, therefore, encourage you to adopt SAMHSA's principles in your work with your clients. Following, we describe how each principle applies to HST.

Principle 1: Safety

SAMHSA's (2014) first principle is safety, meaning that clients should feel safe internally and in the clinical environment. From an HST perspective, clients who have a history of trauma are not good candidates for HST until there is *significant safety in the therapeutic relationship* (Armstrong, 2008). Because HST can be such a powerful approach, clients must have a baseline of safety and trust with the therapist so that they are not overwhelmed with the sandtray process. HST can feel threatening and dangerous to a client with a background of trauma or misattuned attachment even with a solid therapeutic relationship. Therefore, do not attempt sandtray with clients until you are convinced that they can enter an HST experience without being harmed. Of course, there will be times when you thought your client was ready for HST and they become flooded emotionally and are unable to feel regulated. Our suggestion in this case is to back out of HST and focus on grounding and regulation with your client.

In addition, as a humanistic sandtray therapist, you can contribute to an environment of safety by ensuring that you are inclusive of differences in clients' sensory systems, particularly touch. One issue involves the use of therapeutic touch. Although part of the humanistic sandtray therapist's role is to act as co-regulator, we would highly recommend that you avoid engaging in therapeutic touch with clients unless you ask for explicit permission from the client and provide them with your rationale for such touch. We also recommend additional training in the role of touch in the psychotherapeutic relationship. Relatedly, Gonzalo Marrodán and Moraga (2024) suggested that sandtray therapists should be mindful of where they position themselves physically with regard to the client. We agree with their argument that some clients who have experienced trauma may have neuroceptive responses to the therapist's physical proximity during sandtray scene creation and processing. Therefore, we recommend that you check in with your client's here-and-now experiencing of your physical distance from them.

Another issue in terms of safety involves the sand itself. Because clients who have experienced trauma may feel repulsed when they touch certain textures, we recommend that you be prepared to offer a different stratum such as uncooked rice, beans, or even marbles. Some clients may feel safest with an empty tray, too (Homeyer & Lyles, 2022). You may need to take time to explore different textures with your client to discover that which assists them in co-regulation.

Principle 2: Trustworthiness and Transparency

SAMHSA's (2014) second principle refers to practitioners creating a sense of trust with their clients through transparent procedures. In HST, therapists work to create a deeply trusting therapeutic relationship based on Rogers' (1957) core conditions. However, in terms of clarity of procedures, we recommend that you talk openly with your client about the HST process and obtain their voluntary agreement to participate in this approach. One best practice is to provide language in your informed consent about HST. A sample informed consent that you can use and adapt is located in Appendix B at the end of this book.

Principle 3: Peer Support

SAMHSA (2014) recommended that practitioners provide referrals or other opportunities for clients to engage in peer support with other trauma survivors. There are two major ways for you to attend to this principle. One way is to provide updated referral resources for local peer support groups. Another way is to offer an HST group in which trauma survivors create and process sandtrays in a group setting. See Chapter 9 for more about applying HST in group work.

Principle 4: Collaboration and Mutuality

SAMHSA (2014) outlined that "healing happens in relationships and in the meaningful sharing of power and decision-making" (p. 11). This principle is aligned with how humanistic sandtray therapists view not only their therapeutic relationships with clients, but also the entire process of HST. Sandtray is a collaborative approach in which one of the major goals is to bring clients *at choice* through increased awareness and a recognition that clients are in the drivers' seat. Although HST may be more directive at times and more non-directive at others, under a trauma-informed care framework, clients are an integral part of their own healing across the HST process. Humanistic sandtray therapists, like all therapists, can never be in a completely egalitarian relationship with clients; however, they encourage an atmosphere of mutuality and place utmost importance on the therapeutic relationship.

Principle 5: Empowerment, Voice, and Choice

As I (Ryan) discussed in Chapter 2, ensuring you have access to representative miniatures for your client population is an incredibly important part of creating and maintaining a humanistic sandtray collection; it is also one significant way that humanistic sandtray therapists can follow SAMHSA's (2014) fifth principle. In terms of trauma-informed care, having access to various symbols of trauma allows clients to use their voice, feel empowered as they process transitioning from victim identity to survivor identity, and choose how to respond to their trauma reactions. When working with clients who have experienced trauma, following are categories and examples of miniatures that will help clients symbolize their experiences:

- *Self-injury and suicidal ideation*: A knife, rope, gun, figures who are cutting themselves.
- *Substance and behavioral addictions*: Pill bottles, alcohol bottles, syringe, junk food (often found in dollhouse sections at craft stores or at American Girl stores), gym weights.
- *Violence*: Bombs, missiles, tank, drone, military equipment, army helicopter, fighter jet, chain, handcuffs.
- *Abusers and perpetrators*: These are usually figures that are considered to be in the "evil" category, a sheep and wolf, characters who appear devious or as tricksters.

- *Emergency and crisis response*: Police car, SWAT team vehicle, ambulance, hospital building, fire engine, stretcher, medical personnel.

Principle 6: Cultural, Historical, and Gender Issues

Finally, SAMHSA (2014) established a principle regarding cultural competencies, practitioner self-awareness of biases, and meeting clients where they are based on their cultural worldviews. This principle is in line with the American Counseling Association's (2014) code of ethics. Humanistic sandtray therapists serve clients from a non-assumptive position, embracing cultural humility and making efforts to view clients' worlds from the client's perceptual context. You can read more about the HST approach to cultural competency and cultural issues in Chapter 6.

Conclusion

Discoveries regarding the relationship among human beings' psychological dynamics and brain functioning have led to a greater understanding of the impact of psychotherapy on attachment and trauma. By nature, sandtray therapy is an approach that is appropriate for clients who have experienced trauma (Steele & Malchiodi, 2012) because it activates neurophysiological processes that can become dysregulated and provides a therapeutic space for clients to discover new ways to regulate their emotional and reactionary responses. HST is an especially valuable approach for clients with trauma backgrounds because of its emphasis on holism, engaging the client's mind and body. Because humanistic sandtray therapists work in the here and now and focus on exploration, discovery, and awareness, the HST phases, structure, and process, as described in Chapters 3 and 4, can provide a foundation for clients to heal elements of themselves that tend to respond with fear, anxiety, and dysregulation.

References

American Counseling Association. (2014). *Code of ethics*. Author. https://www.counseling.org/resources/aca-code-of-ethics.pdf

Armstrong, S. A. (2008). *Sandtray therapy: A humanistic approach*. Ludic Press.

Badenoch, B. (2008). *Being a brain-wise therapist: A practical guide to interpersonal neurobiology*. Norton.

Damasio, A. (2021). *Feeling and knowing: Making minds conscious*. Pantheon.

Dawson, P. H. (2024). *Sand therapy for out of control sexual behavior, shame, and trauma: Treatment approaches beyond words*. Routledge.

Doidge, N. (2007). *The brain that changes itself: Stories of personal triumph from the frontiers of brain science*. Penguin.

Edelman, G. M., & Tononi, G. (2000). *A universe of consciousness: How matter becomes imagination.* Basic.

Fraser, T. (2022). It is never too late: Healing trauma across the life span with sandtray therapy. In R. Grayson & T. Fraser (Eds.), *The embodied brain and sandtray therapy: Stories of healing and transformation* (pp. 54–70). Routledge.

Gonzalo Marrodán, J. L., & Moraga, R. B. (2024). *Sandtray applications to trauma therapy: A model towards relational harmony.* Routledge.

Grayson, R. (2022). Healing the embodied brain: The neurobiology of sandtray therapy. In R. Grayson & T. Fraser (Eds.), *The embodied brain and sandtray therapy: Stories of healing and transformation* (pp. 28–53). Routledge.

Habib, N. (2019). *Activate your vagus nerve: Unleash your body's ability to heal.* Ulysses.

Hebb, D. O. (1949). *The organization of behavior: A neurophysiological theory.* Wiley.

Heller, L., & LaPierre, A. (2012). *Healing developmental trauma: How early trauma affects self-regulation, self-image, and the capacity for relationship.* North Atlantic.

Homeyer, L. E., & Lyles, M. N. (2022). *Advanced sandtray therapy: Digging deeper into clinical practice.* Routledge.

Kain, K. L., & Terrell, S. J. (2018). *Nurturing resilience: Helping clients move forward from developmental trauma—An integrative somatic approach.* North Atlantic.

Konkel, L. (2018). The brain before birth: Using fMRI to explore the secrets of fetal neurodevelopment. *Environmental Perspectives, 126,* 112001-1-5. https://doi.org/10.1289/EHP2268

Levine, P. A. (2015). *Trauma and memory: Brain and body in a search for the living past: A practical guide for understanding and working traumatic memory.* North Atlantic.

MacLean, P. D. (1990). *The triune brain in evolution: Role in paleocerebral functions.* Springer.

Merzenich, M. M., Tallal, P., Peterson, B., Miller, S., & Jenkins, W. M. (1999). Some neurological principles relevant to the origins of—the cortical plasticity-based remediation of—developmental language impairments. In J. Grafman & Y. Christen (Eds.), *Neuroplasticity: Building a bridge from the laboratory to the clinic* (pp. 169–187). Springer.

Miller-Karas, E. (2015). *Building resilience to trauma: The trauma and community resiliency models.* Routledge.

Perry, B., & Szalavitz, M. (2006). *The boy who was raised as a dog and other stories from a child psychiatrist's notebook: What traumatized children can teach us about loss, love, and healing.* Basic.

Porges, S. W. (2011). *Polyvagal theory: The neurophysiological foundations of emotions, attachment, communication, and self-regulation.* Norton.

Porges, S. W. (2021). Polyvagal theory: A biobehavioral journey to sociality. *Comprehensive Psychoneuroendocrinology, 7,* 1–7. https://doi.org/10.1016/j.cpnec.2021.100069

Rogers, C. R. (1957). The necessary and sufficient conditions of therapeutic personality change. *Journal of Consulting Psychology, 21*(2), 95–103. https://psycnet.apa.org/doi/10.1037/h0045357

Shankar, S. (2016). *How to help your child (and you) break the stress cycle and success-fully engage with life.* Penguin.

Steele, W., & Malchiodi, C. A. (2012). *Trauma-informed practices with children and adolescents.* Routledge.

Substance Abuse and Mental Health Services Administration (SAMHSA) (2014). *Concept of trauma and guidance for a trauma-informed approach.* https://store.samhsa.gov/sites/default/files/sma14-4884.pdf

Waxenbaum, J. A., Reddy, V., & Varacallo, M. (2023). Anatomy, Autonomic Nervous System. StatPearls. https://www.ncbi.nlm.nih.gov/books/NBK539845/

Part II

Developmental Considerations and Cultural Adaptations

Chapter 6

Multicultural Adaptations of Humanistic Sandtray Therapy

Ryan D. Foster, Beck A. Munsey, and Ioana Mărcuș

Humanistic sandtray therapists are bound philosophically to adapting each phase of the HST approach to clients' perceptions of their cultural dynamics. Each client arrives in the consultation room embodying intersectional identities, and humanistic therapists inherently meet the client as they are in the moment. The way in which humanistic sandtray therapists meet their clients can impact the therapeutic relationship as well as clients' abilities to create a scene in the tray that accurately represents who they are and how they perceive themselves, their environment, and their emerging needs. In this chapter, we will discuss multicultural adaptations of HST to account for intersectional identities in the areas of ethnicity and race, socioeconomic status, sexual and affectional orientation, indigenous status, national origin and language, gender, and religion and spirituality. We will review ways in which HST can be used to assist clients in their exploration of cultural self-perceptions, including example sandtray prompts and suggestions on the types of miniatures you can consider including in your collection.

Cultural Humility

Humanistic sandtray therapists adopt a mode of active acceptance of who a client is by operating from a framework of cultural humility, defined as "a process of openness, self-awareness, being egoless, and incorporating self-reflection and critique after willingly interacting with diverse individuals" (Foronda et al., 2016, p. 213). Cultural humility is an integral part of self-work for sandtray therapists (Homeyer & Lyles, 2022). When therapists operate from a place of cultural humility, they are emphasizing "ways of *being with* clients that prioritize and value diverse cultural identities" (Mosher et al., 2017; italics theirs). Humanistic therapists treasure who their clients are and open themselves up to a deep sense of empathic resonance, contact, and inclusion with their clients. In HST, presence inherently includes mutuality and respect for the uniqueness of the other person while

DOI: 10.4324/9781032664996-8

attending to the client's emerging needs. Clients' needs cannot be separated from their cultural context; culture is part of their ground of experiencing. Therapists must remain active in approaching clients with cultural humility in order to advance depth of the therapeutic relationship, a core value in HST. The sand tray is a place to enact cultural humility.

Cultural Differences between the Humanistic Sandtray Therapist and Client

Inevitably, humanistic sandtray therapists will work with clients with whom they differ in one or more aspects of their cultural identities and for whom this difference presents challenges in the therapeutic relationship. HST is an intimate relational experience that requires deep trust and safety between therapist and client. In your journey to become a humanistic sandtray therapist, we encourage you to lean into Rogers' (1957) necessary conditions to be your guide when relational tension arises due to cultural differences. However, Rogers' conditions have a reciprocal relationship with cultural humility practices; therefore, humanistic sandtray therapists should focus on elements of therapeutic practice that provide a safe and open foundation for clients' identities.

Mosher et al. (2017) noted four ways in which therapists can apply cultural humility in their clinical practice: engage in critical self-examination and self-awareness; build the therapeutic alliance; repair cultural ruptures; and navigate value differences. To engage in critical self-examination and self-awareness, Mosher et al. suggested that therapists continually attend to, discover, and arrive at increasing depths of understanding their own biases and culturally intersectional standpoints. In terms of the therapeutic alliance, Mosher et al. encouraged therapists to maintain an inviting presence toward clients' cultural identities. One way that humanistic sandtray therapists can be invitational is to curate miniatures that reflect not only visible singular cultural identities, but also intersectional identities. For example, having miniatures that are people of color who also have a visible ability difference, such as a person who is Black and in a wheelchair. The third focus is on repairing cultural ruptures. Therapists are human beings who create microaggressions in the consultation room from time to time. Sometimes this happens when the therapist makes an inference about a particular miniature in the sandtray scene. Humanistic sandtray therapists own their mistakes, communicate genuinely with clients, and open a conversation to gather feedback from clients. Finally, Mosher et al. discussed ways to navigate value differences such as religion and politics. They suggested that "culturally humble therapists remain other-oriented in that they focus on clients' values more than their own" (p. 228), which mirrors the heart of humanism in counseling and psychotherapy. During HST, therapists are best equipped when they filter out their own preconceptions of the scene in the tray, give up on notions of interpretation, and embody a discovery and exploration system that works alongside their clients.

ADDRESSING Model

Hays (2022) outlined an intersectional model that we integrate in the practice of HST, called ADDRESSING, which stands for **A**ge and generational influences, **D**evelopmental disability or other **D**isability, **R**eligion and spirituality, **E**thnic and racial identity, **S**ES/social class, **S**exual orientation, **I**ndigenous heritage, **N**ational origin, and **G**ender. This model is inclusive of the concept of cultural humility and includes notions of "compassion, veracity, and courage" (p. 16). Hays proposed that best practice is for therapists to examine and retool their personal qualities, self-knowledge, relationship skills, and cultural knowledge in order to engage in culturally responsive care. In this section, we will discuss most of the cultural identities included in the ADDRESSING framework and ways to incorporate them into sandtray work, except for age and generational influences, which are detailed in Chapter 7, and disability, which is detailed in Chapter 8. Those two areas warranted their own chapters due to significant modifications that may need to be made to the HST process when working with those populations. We will examine the remaining identities in the order of the ADDRESSING acronym.

Religious and Spiritual Identities and Experiences

Garrett (2015) noted that clients who seek counseling in secular and nonsecular settings alike may find sandtray to be an appropriate medium through which to explore themes of spirituality, religion, and existential meaning. In our experience, clients often symbolize the place of spirituality in their lives in their trays. They may place figures representing their current spiritual or religious belief system, their relationship to their beliefs, or traumatic experiences related to past spiritual or religious experiences or identities. Foster and Armstrong (2017) defined religion as "a culturally universal social institution that people create to perpetuate doctrine and practice related to spirituality" (p. 133). They further defined spirituality as "an ultimate nature, meaning, and purpose of the universe and, specifically with reference to people, to personal experiences, beliefs, and actions related to an ultimate nature, meaning, and purpose of the universe" (p. 33). Young and Cashwell (2020) noted that spirituality and religion were separate but related concepts. Spiritual and religious identity development is complex and intertwined with other developmental processes, and several models exist that attempt to capture these processes (Foster & Holden, 2020). However, most developmental models tend to lean toward a Western point of view and do not fully incorporate indigenous or

Eastern conceptions of spirituality or religion. Nevertheless, when spirituality or religion is included as ground or figure during a client's sandtray experience, humanistic sandtray therapists certainly need to be prepared to appropriately process these areas. We refer you to Foster and Holden's (2020) summary of spiritual and religious development models to help you feel grounded in these concepts.

Additionally, clients may represent their spiritually transformative experiences in their trays. Pargament (2006) defined spiritual transformation as "a fundamental change in the place of the sacred or the character of the sacred in the life of the individual" (p. 18). According to Pargament, people create their individual framework of "the sacred" as it can refer to a non-theistic or theistic symbol of the divine. Once I (Ryan) had a client represent "the sacred" as a stack of books symbolizing knowledge and she spoke of how continuing to expand her understanding of the world contributed to major shifts in the ways she made meaning. Spiritual transformation can take many different forms in a client's life, as it may lead to changes that lie on continuums of gradual—sudden, regressive—progressive, expected—unexpected, and sought—unsought (Foster & Holden, 2020). HST can assist clients in discovering these elements of spiritual transformation and for those who feel out of control with experiences associated with spiritual transformation, in gaining a sense of empowerment.

Suggested Sandtray Prompts

Although elements of spirituality or religion may show up in a client's sandtray with other prompts, some clients may want to directly explore these areas, particularly if they have unfinished business. Following are some sandtray prompts that we suggest in order to assist in the client's exploration of their spirituality, religion, and related experiences and needs:

- Create a scene that embodies your experience of your own spirituality and/or religion.
- Create a scene that describes the place of spirituality and/or religion in your life.
- Create a scene about the ways in which you make meaning.
- Create a scene that captures how you view the ultimate nature of the universe.
- Create a scene about your experience of spiritual transformation.
- Create a scene about your view and the place of the sacred in your life.

Miniatures

When we think of miniatures to include as part of your collection, the word *numinous* comes to mind. Hopefully, the following objects provide you a launchpad for your collection representing religious and spiritual identities and experiences:

- *Spiritual and/or religious leaders or sages*: Buddha, Jesus Christ, Pillaiyar/ Ganesha and other Hindu gods and goddesses, Christian preachers, Catholic and Hindu priests, imams, nuns, and rabbis. To the best of your ability, ensure that you include visibly diverse religious leaders.
- *Spiritual and/or religious symbols*: Star of David, Christian cross, menorah, Ichthys, Wheel of Dharma, Eye of Horus, Sigel of Baphomet, pentacle, Taijitu ("yin and yang symbol"), Druze star, nine-pointed star, and star and crescent.
- *Spiritual and/or religious experiences*: Sun and moon, rainbow, stormy cloud, tunnel, tornado, waterfall, gemstones of various colors and chakras, people or animals in yoga poses, variety of trees, fire, and stones with meaningful messages or quotes.
- *Spiritual and/or religious buildings or places*: Christian and/or Catholic churches, Notre-Dame, the Taj Mahal, mosques, Stonehenge, a mountain, Ankgor Wat, pyramids, and the Sphinx.

Ethnic and Racial Identities

Although ethnic and racial identities have been salient topics in our field, research and clinical applications are still emergent and struggle to keep pace with the needs of individual clients and clinicians. As clinicians we are interested in how individuals see themselves relative to their cultural beliefs, values, and behaviors; therefore, ethnic identity is the more appropriate construct on which to focus than racial identity. Phinney (1996) developed the multiethnic identity development model, asserting that ethnic identity changes over time, context, and across individuals. Phinney contended that as the individual becomes increasingly aware of discrimination and racism in the context of the larger society, their identity development shifts. This carries important implications for clinical practice and could be an area in which to explore with clients in HST.

In terms of ethnic and racial identity awareness, people who identify as other ethnic groups score higher than people who identify as White, and African Americans score higher than any other group (Phinney, 1996). Ethnic identity and its development have been researched in the context of specific groups, such as Black (Cross, 1991) and White (Helms, 1990); however, Phinney (1996) provided an understanding of its development and process in a larger context. Phinney's model of ethnic identity development consists of three stages. During the initial stage, children and adolescents place little value on influencing their own ethnic identity development and tend to view themselves based on environmental influences, both positive and negative. In the second stage, adolescents engage in an ethnic identity search in which culture and ethnicity become a significant part of self-understanding. In the final stage, which typically takes place during adulthood, the individual achieves a well-defined ethnic identity, and this identity may have varying degrees of importance to their overall sense of self.

HST can be a relevant medium through which clients can explore their ethnic identities and environmental experiences. Sandtray provides a safe space in which clients can explore negative experiences such as microaggressions and oppression as well as positive experiences such as the value that their ethnic identities bring to their lives. HST can also aid in the identity development process. For example, clients in the second stage of Phinney's (1996) model can use HST to reflect on discoveries they have made about the historical elements, values, and present status of their ethnic group. Clients in the final stage could explore how they view their relationships with other ethnicities, particularly the dominant culture, and their emotional reactions to these relationships.

Suggested Sandtray Prompts

Following are some sandtray prompts that we suggest in order to assist in the client's exploration of their ethnic and racial identities and related needs:

- Create two trays. In one tray, create a scene that includes how you experience your various cultural identities. In the other tray, create a scene that includes how you perceive others view your cultural identities.
- Create a scene that embodies your experience of your identity.
- Create a scene of the impact of discrimination and oppression on your life.
- Create a tray that represents your experiences of microaggression.
- Create a tray about how you represent yourself to others in predominately White environments.
- Create a tray about how you represent yourself to others in predominately Black, Indigenous, and people of color (BIPOC) environments.
- Create a tray that represents your perspective on power in your relationships, whether work or personal.
- How would you represent power and privilege in your tray?
- Create a tray about your experiences of power differences within your own culture.

Miniatures

Although having a collection of miniatures representative of all cultural or ethnic groups would be incredibly difficult to curate, we encourage you to attempt to be inclusive of a wide range of skin colors and ethnic backgrounds. If you are working predominantly with a certain group, attaining miniatures representative of this group can be done collaboratively with clients for a more inclusive approach. With these caveats in mind, here are our suggestions in the area of ethnic and racial identities:

- *Diversity in physical appearance*: Miniatures with various skin colors, facial features, and hair textures, colors, and lengths.
- *Diversity in outer wear*: Miniatures aligned with various ethnic and cultural dress.
- *Cultural symbolism, such as miniatures representing cultural leaders*: Dr. Martin Luther King, Harriet Tubman, Gandhi, and other widely recognized figures.
- *Diversity in popular culture*: Popular musicians, artists, athletes, and actors who reflect the client's cultural identity.
- *Cultural symbolism, such liberation symbolism, cultural pride symbolism*: David's star, Japanese cherry trees, Holocaust remembrance, Chinese watercolor art, Torii gates, tree of life.
- *Cultural experiences*: Slavery and its abolition, figures symbolic of the Black Lives Matter movement.

Socioeconomic Status

Socioeconomic status (SES) and social class are neglected oftentimes in both research and clinical work; SES captures income, occupation, and education. Social class is a complex cultural identity that includes SES factors and shapes individuals' worldviews, values, beliefs, and ways of being, accounting for emic and etic individual and group experiences (Cook et al., 2020). SES plays a significant role in access to therapy and is infused in all layers of an individual's life, behaviors, and actions, and oftentimes their mental health outcomes (Giebel et al., 2020). Therefore, HST can act as a vehicle for clients to explore self-understanding in context of how their early experiences shaped their current worldview in terms of issues such as financial stability/instability, power and privilege, economic oppression, food insecurity, and related experiences.

Suggested Sandtray Prompts

Following are some sandtray prompts that we suggest in order to assist in the client's exploration of their socioeconomic status and related needs:

- Create a tray representing your current and/or past experiences of your social class/SES today (e.g., access to food, health care, education, childcare, housing, etc.).

- Create a scene that represents the most salient aspects of your SES challenges.
- Create a tray about your experiences of economic oppression.
- Create a tray about how your childhood SES impacts you now.
- Create a tray capturing how your identities together may impact you (intersectionality).

Miniatures

As you think about adding miniatures representing SES and social class, we recommend that you consider intersectionality as well as polarities of wealth and poverty, privilege and oppression, and vague and specific symbols. Following are some examples of miniatures you may want to consider:

- *Miniatures representing money, class, power, and/or status within various cultures (may be culture specific)*: Dollar bills, credit cards, gold watches, luxury cars.
- *Miniatures representing leaders with high achieved economic status*: Oprah Winfrey, Rihanna, Mark Cuban, Jeff Bezos, Snoop Dogg, other anonymous people who appear wealthy.
- *Miniatures representing presidents or political leaders*: Barack Obama, George Washington, Ronald Reagan, Donald Trump.
- *Experiences that capture the rise or crash of housing market or stock market*: Stock market ticker, "for sale" real estate sign.
- *Representations of poverty*: Homeless person, houses or apartment buildings that appear to be in disrepair.
- *Miniatures representing materialism, capitalism, class, economics, and power*: Mansions, smaller dwellings, high rise buildings, private jets, luxury cars, or other overt or implied symbols of status or lack of status.

Sexual and Affectional Orientation and Identity

Humanistic sandtray therapy can offer a boundaried environment in which clients can explore their sexual and affectional orientation and identities. In this chapter, we use the Society for Sexual, Affectional, Intersex, and Gender Expansive Identities (SAIGE) acronym LGBTGEQIAP+, which stands for **L**esbian, **G**ay, **T**rans, transgender, and Two Spirit (2S; Native Identity), **G**ender **E**xpansive, **Q**ueer and questioning, **I**ntersex, **A**gender, asexual, and aromantic, **P**ansexual, pan/polygender, poly relationship systems, and ± We continue to be Inclusive of Other related identities and committed to ever expanding, learning, and growing the acronym and our understanding of these identities (Ausloos, 2023). It is important to note not all LGBTGEQIAP+ clients come into therapy to work on issues surrounding identity. Many clients who are comfortable with their identities will come into session to work on issues similar to those of heterosexual and cisgender clients. Clients who want to explore their sexual and affectional orientations and identities can benefit greatly from creative and affirming approaches like HST to assist in their identity exploration.

Conceptualizing clients using sexual and affectional orientation identity models is not a one size fits all approach. The research is relatively new on identity models for the LGBTGEQIAP+ community and started in the late 1970s (Bilodeau & Renn, 2005). Many of the identity models have some key similarities: awareness, understanding their identity, finding community in the LGBTGEQIAP+, and incorporating identity into all their identities. Most of the models incorporate a realization of being attracted to members of the same sex or being attracted to someone outside of the binary, and during this realization it is common for clients to deny, try to minimize, or in some cases even reject their identity (Gonsiorek & Weinrich, 1995). The first identity model was created by Cass (1979, 1984). This model focused on gay males and lesbian women. The next model was created by Troiden (1979, 1988) and considered LGBQ identities. In 1991, Falco created a model looking at sexual identity development. Subsequently, D'Augelli (1994) conceptualized the life span and the processes for sexual affections and gender identity. McCarn and Fassinger (1996) presented a lesbian model of the process of individual sexual identity development. Weinberg, Williams, and Pryor (1994) focused their model on bisexuality development, understanding the unique development for bisexual individuals. In HST, we integrate these identity models to conceptualize where our client is in their development and process where they would like to go in their development.

In addition to identity models, humanistic sandtray therapists can be affirming when viewing LGBTGEQIAP+ queer identities and relationships in a positive lens rather than strictly focusing on challenges. Conversely, HST can provide a safe space for clients to address impacts of discrimination, oppression, and homo/trans phobias on the lives of clients. Furthermore, although coming out can be a major milestone for clients as they come to terms with their identity, it is not the job of the humanistic sandtray therapist to decide if a client should come out or not. Clients must weigh their environments, their mental health, and their safety when deciding to come out (Solomon et al., 2018). Some clients may never come out to friends or family, and they may only come out to you, as their safe place. Also, the coming out process is not a one-time event and can be more of a back and forth or fluid process. Some clients may come out in some environments and not in others. For example, a client may perceive more safety in coming out to a group of friends rather than coming out to their immediate family. Humanistic sandtray therapists hold space for clients to include in their trays those environments or individuals to whom they would like to come out.

Suggested Sandtray Prompts

As with other elements of culture, clients' sexual and affectional identities may naturally emerge in open-ended sandtray prompts. However, for clients who express a desire to process their identities, following are some sandtray prompts that we suggest in order to assist in the client's exploration of their sexual and/or affectional orientation(s), identity, and related experiences:

- Create a scene of your feelings around your awareness of your identity today.
- Create a scene that embodies your experience of your LGBTGEQIAP+ identity.
- Create a scene of your experiences of your coming out process.
- Create a scene of the impact of discrimination, oppression, or homo/trans phobias on your life.
- Create a scene that represents how your sexual/affectional identity intersects with your other identities.

Miniatures

In our experiences, clients often need miniatures that represent their sexual and affectional orientations to be able to explore their identities in their trays. Humanistic sandtray therapists who do not have these figures may run the risk of disaffirming clients' needs to explore fully their senses of self. This disaffirmation can be a symbol to the client that the therapist perceives their identity to be unimportant, which can lead to a rift in therapeutic rapport. Following are some miniatures that you should consider including in your collection:

- *Pride colors and symbols*: Miniatures that represent the pride colors of each identity, such as flags, painted rocks, and wooden figures.
- *Diverse couples*: Same-sex miniatures embracing or showing romantic and affectional love.
- *Inclusive families*: Families that have inclusive representation of LGBTGEQIAP+.
- *Bridges painted in pride colors*: Bridges can represent many things for clients processing identities.
- *Intersection of sexual and affectional identity and spirituality and religion:* Spiritual or religious figures in different pride colors.

Indigenous Status

We acknowledge that sand paintings or *iikaah* have been an ancient healing art used by the Navajo community for centuries (Campbell, 1940; Navajo People, n.d.) and they may be part of a religious healing ceremony. Sand painting is sacred and considered a dynamic living entity created by the shaman and the ailing person. Sand paintings are also temporary as they take on the illness and, as a result, must be destroyed. In HST, we attempt to recognize and honor a client's indigenous identity in therapeutic work and how this dimension adds to their strengths and their vulnerability. The indigenous community in the United States has experienced a great degree of trauma and racism, and creating a safe place in the sand tray to capture and represent these kinds of experiences could be powerful (Navajo People, n.d.).

Suggested Sandtray Prompts

Following are some sandtray prompts that we suggest in order to assist in the client's exploration of their indigenous identity and related needs:

- Create a tray about your embodied sense of your (indigenous) identity.
- Create a scene that explores your connection to your indigenous community.
- Create a tray representing your challenges of living in a world dominated by non-indigenous people and environments.
- Create a scene about the place of your voice in the dominant culture.
- Create a scene about your experiences of cultural appropriation or mischaracterization of who you are or your community.
- Create a scene about your experiences of historical or transgenerational trauma.

Miniatures

There are currently 574 federally recognized tribes (BIA, 2023), and a complete representation of every indigenous nation or tribe may not be possible. However, we recommend becoming familiar with the nations inhabiting your area and researching their culture, traditions, wear, and practices, enabling a more accurate representation. Following are examples of miniatures we recommend:

- *Various indigenous groups, including various tribes by dress*: Include groups native to your region.
- *Indigenous leaders*: Powhatan, Crazy Horse, Sitting Bull, Susan La Flesche Picotte, Dennis Banks.
- *Miniatures capturing spiritual and healing practices*: Medicine wheel and four directions, Hohule'a, the Hawai'ian Voyaging Canoe, Medicine Lodges, sacred animals and plants.
- *Indigenous experiences and symbols*: Feathered war bonnets, the bear, the sun, an arrow, a circle.

National Origin and Language

National origin and language are a significant part of a person's identity, particularly if the person is a first-generation immigrant. Generational status and acculturation are strong determinants of cultural maintenance and strong intercultural contact and, in turn, predict a higher level of acceptance in the majority group (Matera, Stefanile, & Brown, 2011). Immigrants and refugees can have a wide variety of experiences depending on their other identities and the intersectionality of these identities. Examples of how intersectionality plays a role in immigrant experiences is sometimes politicized, which creates an additional level of systemic discrimination and trauma. For example, refugees seeking asylum from the Middle East may be reluctantly received by members of the dominant culture compared with war refugees from Ukraine. Legal status, ethnicity, age, gender, religion, and level of education play a significant role in immigrants' or refugees' experiences. As a result, HST can provide an open opportunity to explore many facets of these experiences. As an HST therapist, it is important to be informed of the various systemic challenges facing the immigrant or refugee communities in your area, the political and policy implications at the state and national level, as well as local resources to support clients outside of your therapeutic role.

Suggested Sandtray Prompts

Following are some sandtray prompts that we suggest in order to assist in the client's exploration of their national origin, language, and related needs:

- Create a tray to represent your immigration experience (for first-generation clients).
- Create a tray to represent your identity and your family's identity (for second-generation or bi-cultural clients).
- Create a tray to represent the biggest challenges and successes as an immigrant.
- Create a tray to capture what you miss about your home country.
- Create a tray about your experience of refugee camps and seeking asylum.
- How would you capture the legal challenges you are navigating as an undocumented immigrant?
- Create a tray to capture the sense of belonging to your own culture of origin and/or that of being an American (depending on client's level of acculturation).
- Create a tray to capture the trauma you endured in seeking another home for your family.

- Create a tray of your intergenerational trauma.
- Create a tray of your and your family's resilience.

Miniatures

As you are creating your collection of miniatures to represent experiences of immigrants and refugees, we highly recommend that you familiarize yourself with global current events. For this group of clients, often their lives are driven by forces completely outside of their control. Therefore, having miniatures that can symbolize what is happening in the world that may be impacting your clients or their relatives is essential. Here are our suggestions to begin to establish a collection of miniatures for this population:

- *Miniatures representing people of multiple ethnic backgrounds*: Families, individuals with a variety of facial expressions (e.g., sad, angry, happy), flags from countries around the world.
- *Miniatures representing modern wars and global conflicts*: Tanks, Humvees, rifles, destroyed buildings, medical personnel, armed forces personnel.
- *Miniatures representing immigrant caravans*: Groups of people, trucks, walls, camps, barbed wire.
- *Miniatures representing the United States*: The Statue of Liberty, United States flag, Golden Gate Bridge, Brooklyn Bridge.

Gender Expansive Identities

Gender expansive identities are defined as outside of the binary and cisgender identities and refer to "someone whose gender identity and/or gender expression expands beyond, actively resists, and/or does not conform to the current cultural or social expectation of gender, particularly in relation to male or female" (It Gets Better Project, 2022, para. 1). Gender identity is someone's internal sense of self in relation to their understanding or cultural understanding of male/masculinity, female/felinity, or none (HRC Foundation, n.d.). Gender expression is how a person expresses their gender identity or lack of one. A person's expression can be the clothes they wear, hair styles, make-up, mannerisms, and the like. In the United States, concepts of binary gender identity and cisgender expression are often valued over diverse gender identities and expressions. Also, it is important to note that intersex clients may need to explore gender identity and expression and are often left out of conversations when it comes to gender identity and expression. HST can be a useful and creative tool to help clients take their internalized experiences to explore and express their gender identities in a medium that promotes an affirmative space. However, as with sexual orientation and affectional identities, not all clients who identify as gender expansive will need to process or create scenes in their trays about gender; they may come into the therapeutic space to discuss mental health issues like other cisgender clients.

There are two current identity models for gender expansive identities that focus primarily on transgender clients: a transgender identity model (Morgan & Stevens, 2012) and a transgender development model (Pinto & Moleiro, 2015). However, many of the stages and concepts can be applied to your clients with other gender expansive identities. In the transgender identity model (Morgan & Stevens, 2012), transgender and gender non-conforming (TGNC) individuals typically experience first a disconnect between the mind and body. This process can occur in early childhood. The disconnect is between their gender identity and their expression. They may carry this internal rift with them, hidden in the shadows well beyond adolescence and into adulthood, especially if they experience poor environmental supports. During the next stage, TGNC clients keep their gender identity a secret as they learn to negotiate and manage their identities. They may experience a breaking point where they can no longer live in secret. Those TGNC clients who experience this break move into the last stage in this development model of transition—social, medical, and/or legal. Clients explore what transition means to them and how they would like to transition. For example, clients may change their hair style, clothing, and/or pronouns to match their gender identity (social), look toward hormone affirmative therapy and/or surgical procedures (medical), and/or legally change their name and/or change their gender marker (legal transition). Transition looks unique to each TGNC client. Case Study 6.1 represents an application of HST with a client exploring gender identity.

Case Study 6.1: Brandon

Brandon is a 27-year-old transgender male. He initially came into counseling with symptoms of gender dysphoria. As part of his increased sense of self-awareness during the HST process with me (Beck), Brandon identified as transgender. After his self-discovery, Brandon created a scene to process transition, specifically looking at medical transition steps and the anxiety about taking those steps. Brandon first drew a line down the middle of the tray with his finger in the sand and placed a bridge over the line he created in the middle of the tray. On the left side of the tray, he filled it with symbols of femininity (Brandon's word) and with symbols representing important people in his life, and on the right side were symbols of masculinity and hope. Finally, he placed a figure standing on the top of the bridge that represented him. Through processing his scene, Brandon shared feelings of anxiety about moving forward with his transition and the possibility of losing relationships that were created when others perceived him as a woman. Also, Brandon processed he could no longer live inauthentically and have relationships with others who did not see him as a man. The risk of transition and finding happiness was greater than the risk of losing everyone in his life. By participating in HST, it appeared Brandon was able to understand what he needed to do for himself in his transition process, even if it meant losing relationships. Also, he seemed to feel validated in the necessary next steps of his transition.

The transgender development model (Pinto & Moleiro, 2015) focuses on clients who are wanting to explore transition or clients who are already in the initial stages of transition. In the first step, people feel confusion with their gender identity and seek knowledge and understanding to find a label. In the second step, they begin to explore of their newfound identity. The next step is to explore what transitioning looks like to them and what steps need to happen. The final two steps are embracing their gender identity and experiencing their identity as a part of themselves rather than their only or all-encompassing identity.

Either one of these models integrates well with HST. Humanistic sandtray therapists can follow these models in a gender affirming way to support the difficulties and challenges in understanding gender identity when a client experiences an identity outside of the binary. Humanistic sandtray therapists can be affirming by inviting their clients to create trays that capture experiences of discrimination, oppression, and injustices that clients face at each stage of development or from expressing their gender identity in a congruent and authentic way.

Suggested Sandtray Prompts

Following are some sandtray prompts that we suggest in order to assist in the client's exploration of their gender identity and related needs:

- Create a scene of the disconnection from your gender identity and expression.
- Create a scene that embodies your gender identity.
- Create a scene of your transition process (for clients wanting to transition).
- Create a scene of the safe places and people with whom you can be authentic.

- Create a scene of how your gender identity intersects with your other identities.
- Create a scene of your experiences of discrimination, oppression, or identity phobias.

Miniatures

We strongly recommend that humanistic sandtray therapists curate an inclusive collection of miniatures that affirms identities, expressions, and experiences of clients who identify as gender expansive. Clients often need figures that represent their gender identity and expression to be able to explore their identities in their trays. Access to these kinds of miniatures symbolizes to clients that you are an affirming therapist. Otherwise, if you give a client a sandtray prompt without appropriate symbols, you run the risk of creating a rift in the therapeutic relationship. Following are some examples of miniatures to have as part of your collection:

- *Symbols of gender expansive pride*: Miniatures that represent the gender expansive pride colors of each identity, such as flags, painted rocks, and wooden figures.
- *Expansive pronouns*: Miniatures that represent or have pronouns on them, making sure you have pronouns outside of the binary (e.g., they, them, theirs, ze, hir/zie, hirs/zirs), such as rocks or signs.
- *Intersection of gender expansion and spirituality and religion*: Religious figures in different gender expansive pride colors.
- *Bridges*: Bridges painted in gender expansive colors, which can be deeply representative for clients processing gender identity.
- *Symbols of femininity–masculinity continuum*: Miniatures representing concepts of femininity, masculinity, and other expansive identities.

Conclusion

From our point of view, a humanistic sandtray miniatures collection is incomplete without at least a few figures from each of the cultural identities that Hays (2022) identified in her ADDRESSING model. Even if you do not claim a specialization in any of the areas we discussed in this chapter, it is highly likely that you will counsel clients from across the multicultural spectrum. HST can help clients with diverse identities navigate not only pain and trauma associated with systemic oppression and the impact of power and privilege, but also their own identity development. Requiring therapists to integrate cultural humility, HST is inherently a multicultural approach that can help bridge therapist–client divides of nuanced cultural experiences, worldviews, and values.

References

Ausloos, C. D. (2020). LGBTGEQIAP+ initialism [Infographic]. Society for Sexual, Affectional, Intersex, and Gender Expansive Identities. https://saigecounseling. org/initialism/

Bilodeau, B. L., & Renn, K. A. (2005). Analysis of LGBT identity development models and implications for practice. *New Directions for Student Services*, *111*(111), 25–39. https://doi.org/10.1002/ss.171

Cass, V. C. (1979). Homosexual identity formation: A theoretical model. *Journal of Homosexuality*, *4*(3), 219–235. https://doi.org/10.1300/j082v04n03_01

Cass, V. C. (1984). Homosexual identity formation: Testing a theoretical model. *Journal of Sex Research*, *20*(2), 143–167. https://doi.org/10.1080/002244 98409551214

Campbell, I. (1940). Navajo sandpaintings. *Southwest Review*, *25*(2), 143–150. http://www.jstor.org/stable/43462530

Cook, J. M., Clark, M., Wojcik, K., Nair, D., Baillargeon, T., & Kowalik, E. (2020). A 17-year systematic content analysis of social class and socioeconomic status in two counseling journals. *Counseling Outcome Research and Evaluation*, *11*(2), 104–118. https://doi.org/10.1080/21501378.2019.1647409

Cross, W. E., Jr., Parham, T. A., & Helms, J. E. (1991). The stages of Black identity development: Nigrescence models. In R. L. Jones (Ed.), *Black psychology* (3rd ed., pp. 319–338). Cobb & Henry Publishers.

D'Augelli, A. R. (1994). Identity development and sexual orientation: Toward a model of lesbian, gay, and bisexual development. In E. J. Trickett, R. J. Watts, & D. Birham (Eds.), *Human diversity: Perspectives on people in context* (pp. 312–333). Jossey-Bass.

Falco, K. L. (1991). *Psychotherapy with lesbian clients: Theory into practice*. Brunner/ Mazel.

Foronda, C., Baptiste, D. L., Reinholdt, M. M., & Ousman, K. (2016). Cultural humility: A concept analysis. *Journal of Transcultural Nursing*, *27*, 210–221. http://dx.doi.org/10.1177/1043659615592677

Foster, R. D., & Armstrong, S. A. (2017). On the intersection of spiritual and social-emotional development in children and adolescents. *Journal of Child and Adolescent Counseling*, *3*(3), 132–145. https://doi.org/10.1080/23727 810.2017.1341800

Foster, R. D., & Holden, J. M. (2020). Human and spiritual development and transformation. In C. S. Cashwell & J. S. Young (Eds.), *Integrating spirituality and religion into counseling: A guide to competent practice* (3rd ed., pp. 117–142). American Counseling Association.

Garrett, M. (2015). Bridging the gap: Using sandtray for non-secular counseling issues in secular settings. *American Journal of Contemporary Research*, *5*(5), 16–23. https://www.aijcrnet.com/journals/Vol_5_No_5_October_2015/3.pdf

Giebel, C., Corcoran, R., Goodall, M., Campbell, N., Gabbay, M., Daras, K., Barr, B., Wilson, T., & Kullu, C. (2020). Do people living in disadvantaged circumstances receive different mental health treatments than those from less disadvantaged backgrounds? *BMC Public Health*, *20*(1), 651–651. https://doi.org/ 10.1186/s12889-020-08820-4

Gonsiorek, J. C., & Weinrich, J. D. (1995). Definition and measurement of sexual orientation. *Suicide and Life-Threatening Behavior*, 25(Suppl.), 40–51. https://doi.org/10.1111/j.1943-278X.1995.tb00489.x

Hays, P. A. (2022). *Addressing cultural complexities in counseling and clinical practice: An intersectional approach* (4th ed.). American Psychological Association. https://doi.org/10.1037/0000277-000

Helms, J. E. (Ed.). (1990). *Black and White racial identity: Theory, research, and practice*. Greenwood Press.

Homeyer, L. E., & Lyles, M. N. (2022). *Advanced sandtray therapy: Digging deeper into clinical practice*. Routledge. https://doi.org/10.4324/9781003095491

Human Rights Campaign (HRC) Foundation. (n.d.). Sexual orientation and gender identity definitions. Human Rights Campaign. https://www.hrc.org/resources/sexual-orientation-and-gender-identity-terminology-and-definitions

It Gets Better Project. (2022). LGBT+ glossary. https://itgetsbetter.org/glossary/gender-nonconforming/

Matera, C., Stefanile, C., & Brown, R. (2011). The role of immigrant acculturation preferences and generational status in determining majority intergroup attitudes. *Journal of Experimental Social Psychology*, 47(4), 776–785. https://doi.org/10.1016/j.jesp.2011.03.007

McCarn, S. R., & Fassinger, R. E. (1996). Revisioning sexual minority identity formation: A new model of lesbian identity and its implication. *The Counseling Psychologist*, 24, 508–534. https://doi.org/10.1177/0011000096243011

Morgan, S. W., & Stevens, P. E. (2012). Transgender identity development as represented by a group of transgendered adults. *Issues in Mental Health Nursing*, 33(5), 301–308. https://doi.org/10.3109/01612840.2011.653657

Mosher, D. K., Hook, J. N., Captari, L. E., Davis, D. E., DeBlaere, C., & Owen, J. (2017). Cultural humility: A therapeutic framework for engaging diverse clients. *Practice Innovations*, 2(4), 221–233. https://doi.org/10.1037/pri0000055

Navajo People (n.d.). Sand painting. https://navajopeople.org/navajo-sand-painting.htm

Pargament, K. I. (2006). The meaning of spiritual transformation. In J. D. Koss-Chioino & P. Hefner (Eds.), *Spiritual transformation and healing: Anthropological, theological, neuroscientific, and clinical perspectives* (pp. 10–24). Altamira.

Phinney, J. S. (1996). Understanding ethnic diversity: The role of ehnic identity. *American Behavioral Scientist*, 40(2), 143–152. https://doi.org/10.1177/0002764296040002005

Pinto, N., & Moleiro, C. (2015). Gender trajectories: Transsexual people coming to terms with their gender identities. *Professional Psychology: Research and Practice*, 46(1), 12–20. https://doi.org/10.1037/a0036487

Rogers, C. R. (1957). The necessary and sufficient conditions of therapeutic personality change. *Journal of Consulting Psychology*, 21(2), 95–103. https://psycnet.apa.org/doi/10.1037/h0045357

Solomon, D. T., Reed, O. M., Sevecke, J. R., O'Shaughnessy, T., & Acevedo-Polakovich, I. D. (2018). Expert consensus on facilitating the coming-out process in sexual minority clients: A Delphi study. *Journal of Gay & Lesbian Mental Health*, 22(4), 348–371. https://doi.org/10.1080/19359705.2018.1476279

Troiden, R. R. (1979). Becoming homosexual: A model of gay identity acquisition. *Psychiatry: Journal for the Study of Interpersonal Processes*, *42*(4), 362–373. https://doi.org/10.1080/19359705.2018.1476279

Troiden, R. R. (1988). Homosexual development. *Journal of Adolescents Health Care*, *9*(2), 105–113. https://doi.org/10.1016/0197-0070(88)90056-3

U. S. Department of the Interior Indian Affairs (BIA). (2023). Tribal Leaders Directory. https://www.bia.gov/service/tribal-leaders-directory

Weinburger, M. S., Williams, C. J., & Pryor, D. W. (1994). *Dual attraction: Understanding bisexuality*. Oxford University Press.

Young, J. S., & Cashwell, C. S. (2020). Integrating spirituality and religion into counseling: An introduction. In C. S. Cashwell & J. S. Young (Eds.), *Integrating spirituality and religion into counseling: A guide to competent practice* (3rd ed., pp. 3–30). American Counseling Association.

Chapter 7

Humanistic Sandtray Therapy with Preadolescents and Young Adolescents

Thus far, I have discussed HST as a powerful model of sandtray therapy for older adolescents and adults. However, sandtray therapy has strong roots in child psychotherapy and counseling. Lowenfeld (2007) originally developed her World Technique for use with young children and, from a historical point of view, could be considered the earliest example of child-centered expressive therapy, predating even Virginia Axline's (1986) seminal work in what would become known as child-centered play therapy (CCPT). Some clinicians have a sand tray available for use as part of their typical play therapy room setup (Smelser, 2021) with children 3 years old to around functional age 9, referred to as sandtray play therapy (Homeyer & Lyles, 2022). Sandtray can be used as one of many expressive arts protocols with preadolescents (Geldard, Geldard, & Yin Foo, 2018). In addition to its use alongside other expressive arts activities, I suggest that HST is appropriate as a singular approach to psychotherapy and counseling with preadolescents beginning at functional age 10, much like CCPT with younger children (Landreth, 2023). I use the term *functional age* to indicate that one's chronological age is approximately congruent with one's typical holistic developmental capacities (Guralnik & Melzer, 2002). In this chapter, I will discuss the rationale for and adaptations of HST with preadolescents and young adolescents ages 10 to 14 years old.

Rationale for HST with Preadolescents and Young Adolescents

Generally, sandtray therapy is suited uniquely for working with preadolescent and young adolescent clients because of its flexible application to a wide variety of presenting issues as well as its non-reliance on client verbalization of their internal worlds (Armstrong, Foster, & Hickman, 2022; Homeyer & Sweeney, 2023). HST's emphasis on putting the client in the lead and person-centered qualities of the therapeutic relationship, which can promote safety, makes it a good match for working with preadolescents

DOI: 10.4324/9781032664996-9

and young adolescents. In addition, the HST process of exploration and discovery are aligned with preadolescents' and young adolescents' developmental tasks (Armstrong et al., 2022). When therapists are considering using HST with preadolescents and young adolescents, they need a good rationale. Although sandtray is an accepted practice with child, preadolescent, and adolescent clients (Homeyer & Sweeney, 2023), therapists should be intentional in their decision to use it based on clients' unique contexts. There are three main factors to consider: the client's developmental functioning, format of therapy (e.g., individual, group, or family), and therapeutic goals (Geldard et al., 2018).

Developmental Functioning

For functionally aged preadolescents and young adolescents, ages 10 to 14 bring them from a period of relative developmental stability (Ojiambo & Taylor, 2016) to internal chaos (Armstrong et al., 2022). Ojiambo and Taylor (2016) suggested that sandtray therapy based on Oaklander's (2006) gestalt model is clinically appropriate starting at age 10 due to a cross-section of developmental factors. In this section, I will focus on cognitive, psychosocial, and social-emotional developmental factors that make HST a fit for clinical work with preadolescents and young adolescents.

Cognitive Development

Children who are between ages 10 and 12 are making their way toward abstract reasoning but are not quite there yet, cognitively speaking. According to Piaget, preadolescents are transitioning from concrete operations to formal operations (Berk, 2017). During concrete operations, children make decisions based on logical facts that are borne out of their experiences of reality. They are open to taking on new experiences but see the world as an objective place where the "right" way to do things exists, so their failures are compared against an external standard. Around 12 years old, preadolescents begin to enter formal operations, and this will last through adulthood. At this functional age, people can begin to envision a future and make plans for it, reflecting some ability for abstract reasoning; however, it is still tied to logic. In addition, they begin to process verbally thoughts and feelings and can form some language around expressing what is happening internally. However, they tend to experience emotions and thoughts quite concretely. Even during young adolescence, clients can fool therapists into thinking they are more cognitively mature than they really are—they have an emerging, strong hold on language but often struggle with immersion into full abstraction of ideas.

In my experience, preadolescent and young adolescent clients work hard to substantiate their emotional responses based on a perceived factual, concrete circumstance. For example, in therapy, I have found it typical for preteens and young teens to talk more about *why* they feel a certain way based on an event. By 12 years old, they are quite talented at storytelling, and a 13- or 14-year-old will give the therapist a run for their money! Stories are a way that they can symbolize what is going on inside for them. This penchant for metaphor is what can make sandtray such a useful medium for preadolescents (Geldard et al., 2018). Metaphor is an important part of meaning-making and acts to connect a client's inner experiences as well as test out ideas (Mortola, 2006).

Psychosocial Development

According to Erikson's psychosocial stages of development, preteens are working through industry versus inferiority, with some 12-year-olds entering identity versus role confusion (Berk, 2017). During industry versus inferiority, preadolescents become rather aware of their peers and engage in comparison globally, from the decisions that they make to the way that they look. They try on new learned behaviors, some of which become habits for living over the longer term. For example, it is typical for children to learn how to respond to their own emotional experiencing based on what they have learned from others who are important to them. Humanistic sandtray therapists with keen observational skills can attend to these habits of their preadolescent clients. HST can help preteens successfully complete developmental tasks associated with industry versus inferiority resulting in more fulfilling self-concepts to assist them in progressing to the next psychosocial development stage.

Some 12-year-olds are on the cusp of identity versus role confusion, and certainly by the time they are 14 years old they are plodding their way through making sense of themselves by taking more risks; therefore, they start to examine their values, resulting in choices based on their conclusions about what they think is right and wrong (Berk, 2017). They may be able to engage in some self-reflection. It is the beginning of a very long period of self-examination and chaotic expression of who they believe themselves to be or who they wish they were. However, it is likely that when 12-year-old clients present to psychotherapy, they have yet to resolve earlier psychosocial developmental tasks (Broderick & Blewitt, 2019). HST can provide a corrective experience designed to facilitate developmental progression.

Social-Emotional Development

Preadolescents form the capacity for emotionally differentiated thinking (Greenspan & Shanker, 2004). They are beginning to discover cause and effect of environment and emotions. They discover they feel sad when they are left out when their friends get together without them, and they understand the connection between the event and their disappointment. They begin to see the power of social groups as they focus on developing self and a sense of belonging. Some preteens have an easier time than others fitting in with a social group that has an unspoken set of membership rules and roles. HST is a suitable developmental match for encouraging emotionally differentiated thinking because preadolescents can observe concretely patterns of their reactions to their situations and environments. The sand tray gives them a way to examine interactions between person and environment as well as how their sense of group belonging impacts how they view self.

Young adolescents begin developing an "ability to reflect by using an expanding internal standard and a growing internal sense of self encompasses new learning experiences, including physical changes, sexuality, romance and closer, more intimate peer relationships" (Greenspan & Shanker, 2004, p. 81). However, at 13 or 14 years old, therapists often observe teenagers oscillating between a newfound, solid sense of self and an earlier self that seems underdeveloped. One reason is that young adolescents' cognitive abilities tend to change rapidly during this time and are somewhat unstable, so they find comfort in thinking about the world in a concrete fashion. HST can accommodate these rapid shifts from complex to simple ways of feeling, thinking, and behaving, as sandtray allows clients to create scenes that are linear or abstract—metaphor and symbolism remain steadfast pieces of the sandtray experience through this internally chaotic time for young teenagers.

Format of Therapy

Expressive therapies such as sandtray are well suited for both individual and group formats (Homeyer & Sweeney, 2023; Pearson & Wilson, 2009). Armstrong et al. (2017) and Armstrong et al. (2022) noted that HST works well in both individual and group formats for preadolescents and young adolescents. Because preteens and young teens begin to develop self in context of their peers, group HST can be an especially beneficial format (Shen & Armstrong, 2008). I discuss humanistic sandtray group therapy in Chapter 9 of this text.

Therapeutic Goals

The overall goal in working with preadolescents using HST is the same as when therapists work with adolescents or adults. Oaklander (2015) stated that "[m]y goal is to help the child become aware of herself and her existence in her world" (p. 57). Many therapists work with preadolescents in environments such as schools or agency settings that demand efficient outcomes based on behavioral goals. Behavioral goals do not conflict inherently with awareness and humanistic models of care. In HST, therapists assume that behavior will change because increased awareness allows preadolescents to view more choices for relating to their environment. Moreover, Geldard et al. (2018) argued that the use of sandtray could assist in achieving several general goals common to therapeutic work with preadolescents: to gain mastery over current and past unfinished business; to experience empowerment and control of themselves and their immediate environment through experimentation; to express emotions; to learn how to take risks and change behaviors; to advance communication abilities; and to gain increased understanding of self, others, the world, and events in their lives. Therefore, HST is well suited to help clients move toward their psychotherapy goals. When working with preadolescents and young adolescents, humanistic sandtray therapists must adapt how they implement their process skills and relational dynamics to mirror the client's developmental needs.

Adaptations of HST with Preadolescents and Young Adolescents

Humanistic sandtray therapists must be mindful in their work with preadolescents and young adolescents. Even though the ages of children and teens I discuss in this chapter are too old for standard CCPT (Ray, 2016), I would highly recommend that any therapist who works with preadolescents gets training in child-centered or gestalt play therapy. The kinds of dynamics on which play therapists learn to focus, such as observation of client non-verbals and staying within the metaphor, maintain significance in clinical work with preadolescents. For working with preadolescents and young adolescents, Oaklander's (2015) gestalt sandtray process is a developmentally responsive adaptation that aligns with philosophical undercurrents of HST. Before I review application of Oaklander's process to HST, I will offer some concrete tips for having inclusive miniatures. I will also highlight unique features of the therapeutic relationship with preadolescent and young adolescent clients.

Sandtray Miniatures for Preadolescents and Young Adolescents

Humanistic sandtray therapists' collections of miniatures should be inclusive for the client populations with which they work. For preteens and young teens, sandtray therapists should have miniatures that represent characters from popular movies and television shows (Hunter, 2008), comic books including manga, video games, and books. I would encourage therapists to consider including miniatures of important cultural or historical figures as well; for example, having a Ruth Bader Ginsburg figure could mean a lot for a young adolescent who is developing interests in women's rights. Additionally, having fictional characters that may represent younger parts of clients—Sesame Street and Disney miniatures, for example—can be powerful symbols. Also, it is useful to include miniatures that symbolize social interests and activities. Examples include sports miniatures and athletes, musical instruments, books, an artist's palette, skateboards, and a 20-sided roleplaying game die. Finally, I recommend having miniatures that represent problems or issues in a client's life like self-harm, drug and alcohol use, loneliness, friendship, abuse, and school.

The Therapeutic Relationship with Preadolescents and Young Adolescents

Establishing and maintaining a safe therapeutic relationship with preadolescents and young adolescents requires nuances that are different from working with adult clients. Engaging therapeutically with clients during these mystifying developmental periods can be puzzling and sometimes frustrating (Sommers-Flanagan & Sommers-Flanagan, 2007). There are two concepts that drive humanistic sandtray therapists' active participation in the therapeutic relationship with preteens and teens: the relationship triangle (Mortola, 2011) and developmentally responsive authenticity.

The Relationship Triangle

Mortola (2011) described Oaklander's relationship triangle as consisting of the therapist, the sentient client, and the emerging client. The sentient client is the one "who sits before [the therapist] and is aware of [themselves] to some extent" (p. 341). In HST, therapists develop a relationship with the sentient part of the client through aspects of the therapeutic relationship that I discussed in Chapter 1, including good contact and full presence. The emerging client consists of "the parts of the client that the client has not necessarily differentiated, been aware of, or been in contact with" (p. 342). Oaklander's use of expressive arts, including sandtray, was the medium through which the therapist was able to facilitate contact between the salient client with the emerging client. In HST, the therapist focuses on level three and level four metaphor work to open a dialogue between the client's salient and emerging parts. For example, for a client who has created a scene filled with astronauts, spaceships, and aliens, the therapist might ask the client to have a conversation between an astronaut and an alien, both from a first-person point of view. Humanistic sandtray therapists invite their clients into this relational triangle because the therapeutic relationship is the vessel in which here-and-now awareness and paradoxical change occur.

Authenticity

Authenticity, or genuineness, is a core concept of the therapeutic relationship (Rogers, 1957). Authenticity is central to an adolescent's friendships (Damon, 1983; Furman, 1996; Impett et al., 2008; Selman, 1980; Tolman et al., 2006; Tolman & Porche, 2000), mentorships (Spencer, 2006), self-understanding (Ullman, 1987), and therapeutic relationships (Davidson, 2012; Holliman & Foster, 2016). However, therapists who work with preteens and adolescents need to also be *believable* (Holliman & Foster, 2016; Lambert & Barley, 2001; Rogers, 1957)—in other words, clients of this age seem to have a rather astute bullshit detector inherent to their developmental phases. A therapist can send genuine signals of care, but there are ways that can make this seem more believable and congruent than not to this age of clients.

Holliman and Foster (2016) summarized ways in which therapists can more intentionally pursue communication of authenticity to their adolescent clients. Personal confidence of the therapist is one component. When therapists have done their own personal work to perceive themselves as enough both as person and as therapist, they feel freer to be authentically present with clients (Rogers, 1961). Humanistic sandtray therapists can better attune to their authentic presence with clients when they believe in themselves as an important part of client healing. A second component of skillfully embodying authenticity with adolescents is called dissipating tension (Holliman & Foster, 2016), defined as "an authentic way of responding to the underlying and often unspoken issues that exist in the relationship" (p. 64). Dissipating tension begins with the therapist's intentional efforts to really get what is happening for the client from the client's point of view without allowing the therapist's own contact boundary disturbances to get in the way. Humanistic sandtray therapists ought not give in to the kind of therapy that serves only to assuage parents' concerns or goals and to act as a "fixer."

Two practical ways of dissipating tension are to facilitate the client's investment in the process and engage in nest building (Holliman & Foster, 2016). To invite clients into investment in the process of therapy, therapists should seek feedback as this has been found to positively impact treatment outcome (Harmon et al., 2007). For example, therapists who explore their adolescent clients' perceptions about why they are in therapy can better empathically attune to their clients. Adolescents are essentially involuntary clients most of the time, brought there because their parents want therapists to fix them. Humanistic sandtray therapists could investigate clients' perceptions by inviting them to build a sandtray scene based on the prompt, "Create a scene about what your parents (or caregivers) told you about why you're coming here today." A close colleague of mine once told me about his experience as a teenager going to therapy for the first time. His parents took him straight to therapy after coming home from summer camp without advance notice that this would be happening. I often think about how enlightening it would have been if he had created a sandtray based on that experience!

Nest building involves creating an environment that is welcoming and safe to preteens and teenagers (Holliman & Foster, 2016). Thankfully, humanistic sandtray therapists inherently have such an environment with a good sand tray setup. The miniatures on the shelves seem to naturally draw many young clients into the inherent safety of metaphor and symbol. What is important here is to have miniatures that represent all potential aspects of a client's experiencing. Therapists who limit themselves to positive imagery with their sandtray collection are communicating that only certain feelings are allowed here. On the other hand, for a while I had a sandtray collection that leaned in the opposite direction, and I had an "aha" moment that I had more darkness than light in my miniatures collection, so I had to focus on balancing the kinds of symbols I offered my clients. Remaining intentional in communicating authenticity with preadolescent and young adolescent clients can be challenging and altogether rewarding—it is so worth it because it can impact clients' reciprocal transparency in the creation and processing of their trays.

The Process of HST with Preadolescents and Young Adolescents

Humanistic sandtray therapists can provide a more effective space for preteens and teens to engage in HST not only through attending to nuances of the therapeutic relationship but also to concrete ways in which to facilitate sandtray sessions. Mortola (2006) described four phases of expressive therapies based on Oaklander's approach with children and adolescents. The first phase is imaginative experience in which clients are invited into a relaxation and/or guided imagery exercise. As in HST with older adolescents and adults, I recommend that therapists invite clients into a centering experience in order to connect clients to inner experiencing. Preteens and teens have the capability to engage in centering; however, at times they may resist this experience due to feelings of embarrassment. As I discussed in Chapter 4, allow the client to have their experience and never force them to center if they are not open to it.

The second phase in Oaklander's four-phase process is sensory expression (Mortola, 2006). This captures the creation phase of HST. One adaptation for preadolescents and young adolescents is to use Oaklander's basic tray creation prompt:

I would like you to make a scene in the sand. You can use any of the objects you see here, and if there is something you don't see, ask me—maybe I have it. Your scene doesn't have to make sense, or it can. You can choose things because you like them and want to use them. Or you might want to make something special. It can be real or imaginary or like a dream. Anything.

(p. 158)

In addition, Oaklander might provide a child client with a more directive prompt, such as, "Do a scene representing the divorce in your family" (p. 158). Other options for scene creation prompts might shift attention to a typical preadolescent's world of school, peer relationships, self-concept, and body image. Moreover, Fried, McKenna, and Short (2020) provided an example prompt that can be used to explore polarities such as weak/strong, alone/together, brave/afraid, aggressive/passive, and superior/inferior: "Make a scene that is serious, then one that is silly" (p. 57). Preadolescents and young adolescents typically create their scenes in 5 to 10 minutes or less (Armstrong et al., 2022). I have seen several 13-year-old clients create scenes in 90 seconds when they are familiar with the process.

HST integrates Oaklander's third and fourth steps in the processing phase. The third step in Oaklander's process is narrative/metaphoric description (Mortola, 2006) and takes place as therapists engage the client in experiments like enactment and other ways of working with metaphor, as described in Chapter 4 of this text. Oaklander's fourth step, sense-making articulation, applies as the therapist facilitates personalizing the metaphor. During the processing phase of HST, therapists should adjust their facilitative skills to match the developmental level of their individual clients. One issue that sometimes arises when working with preadolescents and young adolescents is their capacity for staying in emotions. They typically have a lower level of tolerance developmentally for being in their feelings in the here and now (Armstrong, 2008). Humanistic sandtray therapists should also expect to respond more frequently to non-verbal expressions of emotion, as clients are learning the language of complex or opposing emotions.

Preadolescents and young adolescents tend to bring in defenses and resistance not only because of their developmental tasks of wanting to experience a sense of belonging even in the therapeutic relationship and to avoid appearing wounded, but also due to histories of hurt and trauma. Oaklander (2006) saw it "as their way of attempting to cope and survive and make contact with the world as best as they can" (p. 23). This concept of resistance differs little from how humanistic sandtray therapists view it in adult clients. However, children's behavioral expressions of resistance are often the very thing that gets them in trouble at school and at home, which makes it meaningful for humanistic sandtray therapists to meet the client where they are at holistically, including their defenses. For example, I used to oversee an HST program for seventh graders in a local middle school. Some of the clients would refuse to even go to the sandtray room with their counseling intern. When this would come up in clinical supervision, I would tell my interns that when a client gives a very clear refusal to do something, meeting them where they are meant respecting their "No, I don't want to go to sandtray today." Relatedly, some clients would create a tray and talk about anything but what was in the scene. For these clients, to gently redirect to the tray while honoring their resistance, I might say something like, "I noticed today you created your scene and wanted to talk about something else. Unless I'm missing something. I wonder if you might tell me something about your scene." A couple of possibilities are that the client experienced a figure emerge that had nothing to do with their scene or they wanted to guard or avoid what the tray ignited in them. In either case, my intention is to meet the client where they are with their resistance to respect and work with it.

Conclusion

HST can be valuable in counseling preadolescent and young adolescent clients because it can be adapted to meet their developmental needs. Oaklander (2015) provided a model of gestalt therapy that works well with preteens and young teens, and I recommend you read her work to deeply familiarize yourself with her process because it translates well to HST. In addition, when humanistic sandtray therapists bring authenticity to their therapeutic relationships with this population, clients will be more apt to engage in the HST process.

References

Armstrong, S. A., Foster, R. D., & Hickman, D. (2022). Humanistic sandtray with preadolescent groups. In C. Mellenthin, J. Stone, & R. J. Grant (Eds.), *Implementing play therapy with groups: Contemporary issues in practice* (pp. 26–38). Routledge.

Armstrong, S. A., Foster, R. D., Brown, T., & Davis, J. (2017). Humanistic sandtray therapy with children and adults. In E. S. Leggett & J. N. Boswell (Eds.), *Directive play therapy: Theories and techniques* (pp. 217–253). Springer.

Axline, V. (1986). *Dibs: In search of self.* Ballantine.

Berk, L. E. (2017). *Development through the lifespan* (7th ed.). Pearson.

Broderick, P., & Blewitt, P. (2019). *The life span: Human development for helping professionals* (5th ed.). Pearson.

Damon, W. (1983). *Social and personality development: Infancy through adolescence.* Norton.

Davidson, M. (2012). "You have to have the relationship": A youth perspective on psychotherapy and the development of a therapeutic relationship (Doctoral dissertation). Simon Fraser University, Burnaby, British Columbia, Canada.

Fried, K., McKenna, C., & Short, S. (2020). *Healing through play—Using the Oaklander model: A guidebook for therapists and counselors working with children, adolescents and families*. Author.

Furman, W. (1996). The measurement of friendship perceptions: Conceptual and methodological issues. In W. M. Bukowski, A. F. Newcomb, & W. W. Hartup (Eds.), *The company they keep: Friendships in childhood and adolescence* (pp. 41–65). Cambridge University Press.

Geldard, K., Geldard, D., & Yin Foo, R. (2018). *Counseling children: A practical introduction* (5th ed.). Sage.

Greenspan, S. I., & Shanker, S. G. (2004). *The first idea: How symbols, language, and intelligence evolved from our primate ancestors to modern humans*. Da Capo Press.

Guralnik, J. M., & Melzer, D. (2002). Chronological and functional ageing. In J. R. M. Copeland, M. T. Abou-Saleh, & D. G. Blazer (Eds.), *Principles and practice of geriatric psychiatry* (2nd ed., pp. 71–74). Wiley.

Harmon, S. C., Lambert, M. J., Smart, D. M., Hawkins, E., Nielsen, S. L., Slade, K., & Lutz, W. (2007). Enhancing outcome for potential treatment failures: Therapist–client feedback and clinical support tools. *Psychotherapy Research*, *17*(4), 379–392. https://doi.org/10.1080/10503300600702331

Holliman, R. P., & Foster, R. D. (2016). Embodying and communicating authenticity in adolescent counseling. *Journal of Child and Adolescent Counseling*, *2*(1), 61–76. https://doi.org/10.1080/23727810.2016.1160353

Homeyer, L. E., & Lyles, M. N. (2022). *Advanced sandtray therapy: Digging deeper into clinical practice*. Routledge. https://doi.org/10.4324/9781003095491

Homeyer, L. E., & Sweeney, D. S. (2023). *Sandtray therapy: A practical manual* (4th ed.). Routledge. https://doi.org/10.4324/9781003221418

Hunter, L. B. (2008). Movie metaphors in miniature: Children's use of popular hero and shadow figures in sandplay. In L. C. Rubin (Ed.), *Popular culture in counseling, psychotherapy, and play-based interventions* (pp. 141–161). Springer.

Impett, E. A., Sorsoli, L., Schooler, D., Henson, J. M., & Tolman, D. L. (2008). Girls' relationship authenticity and self-esteem across adolescence. *Developmental Psychology*, *44*, 722–733. https://doi.org/10.1037/0012-1649.44.3.722

Lambert, M., & Barley, D. E. (2001). Research summary on the therapeutic relationship and psychotherapy outcome. *Psychotherapy*, *38*, 357–361. https://doi.org/10.1037/0033-3204.38.4.357

Landreth, G. L. (2023). *Play therapy: The art of the relationship* (4th ed.). Routledge. https://doi.org/10.4324/9781003255796

Lowenfeld, M. (2007). *Understanding children's sandplay: Lowefeld's World Technique*. Sussex Academic Press.

Mortola, P. (2006). *WindowFrames: Learning the art of gestalt play therapy the Oaklander way*. The Gestalt Press.

Mortola, P. (2011). You, me, and the parts of myself I'm still getting to know: An interview with Violet Oaklander on the role of the relational triangle in her approach to therapeutic work with children and adolescents. In R. G. Lee &

N. Harris (Eds.), *Relational child, relational brain: Development and therapy in childhood and adolescence* (pp. 339–348). The Gestalt Press.

Oaklander, V. (2006). *Hidden treasure: A map to the child's inner self.* Routledge.

Oaklander, V. (2015). *Windows to our children* (35th anniversary ed.). The Gestalt Journal Press.

Ojiambo, D., & Taylor, L. (2016). The extraordinary 10-year-old. In D. C. Ray (Ed.), *A therapist's guide to child development: The extraordinarily normal years* (pp. 136–151). Routledge.

Pearson, M., & Wilson, H. (2009). *Using expressive arts to work with mind, body and emotions.* Jessica Kingsley.

Ray, D. C. (2016). Developmentally appropriate interventions. In D. C. Ray (Ed.), *A therapist's guide to child development: The extraordinarily normal years* (pp. 14–26). Routledge.

Rogers, C. R. (1957). The necessary and sufficient conditions of therapeutic personality change. *Journal of Consulting Psychology, 21*(2), 95–103. https://psycnet.apa.org/doi/10.1037/h0045357

Rogers, C. R. (1961). *On becoming a person.* Houghton Mifflin.

Selman, R. (1980). *The growth of interpersonal understanding.* Academic Press.

Shen, Y., & Armstrong, S. (2008). Impact of group sandtray therapy on the self-esteem of young adolescent girls. *Journal for Specialists in Group Work, 33*(2), 118–137. https://doi.org/10.1080/01933920801977397

Smelser, Q. K. (2021). Exploring gender and sexuality using play therapy. In E. Gil & A. A. Drewes (Eds.), *Cultural issues in play therapy* (2nd ed., pp. 90–110). Guilford Press.

Sommers-Flanagan, J., & Sommers-Flanagan, R. (2007). *Tough kids, cool counseling: User-friendly approaches with challenging youth* (2nd ed.). American Counseling Association.

Spencer, R. (2006). Understanding the mentoring process between adolescents and adults. *Youth and Society, 37*(3), 287–315. https://doi.org/10.1177/0743558405278263

Tolman, D. L., & Porche, M. V. (2000). The Adolescent Femininity Ideology Scale: Development and validation of a new measure for girls. *Psychology of Women Quarterly, 24*, 365–376. https://doi.org/10.1111/pwqu.2000.24.issue-4

Tolman, D. L., Impett, E. A., Tracy, A. J., & Michael, A. (2006). Looking good, sounding good: Femininity ideology and adolescent girls' mental health. *Psychology of Women Quarterly, 30*, 85–95. https://doi.org/10.1111/pwqu.2006.30.issue-1

Ullman, C. (1987). From sincerity to authenticity: Adolescents' views of the "true self." *Journal of Personality, 55*(4), 583–595. https://doi.org/10.1111/jopy.1987.55.issue-4

Chapter 8

Adaptations of Humanistic Sandtray Therapy for People with Disabilities

Ryan D. Foster, Robin Elkins, and James Turnage

In this chapter, we are going to discuss a topic that writers and practitioners have discussed infrequently in sandtray therapy literature historically: people diagnosed with disabilities. We will talk about ability differences that have their roots in genetics as well as acquired differences. Unfortunately, we will only be touching the surface of how to apply HST with clients who arrive to counseling or psychotherapy with these differences. Of note here is our use of the term *disability* and the context of ableism that surrounds this concept. According to Shew (2023), "disability is a social construct—a mismatch between the self and a world that was designed to cater to normative bodies and minds" (p. 21), referring to the social model of disability. Shew noted that the term disability "simply means diverging abilities—*differences*" (p. 28; italics hers). Following Shew's recommendation, we use *disability* throughout this chapter as a global term that refers to it as a social construct rather than using it according to a medical model. This use fits with HST as a non-pathologizing approach. However, in keeping with professional nomenclature, we will also refer to *DSM-5-TR* (American Psychiatric Association, 2022) diagnostic categories. Our major aim is to explore practical ways that HST can be used with clients who have developmental delays, neurodevelopmental diagnoses such as autism spectrum disorder (ASD), and intellectual and developmental disabilities (IDD), as well as those who have inborn or acquired physical disabilities. We will discuss having an inclusive set of miniatures, considerations for accessible sandtray spaces, and using HST when counseling clients in in-home or group home settings.

Our Stories

Before we discuss sandtray adaptations, we want to provide you with some understanding about why facilitating HST alongside people with disabilities is so meaningful for each one of us. Our individual stories provide a roadmap that has led us to feel a strong connection with serving this population of clients. Psychotherapists are often driven to this helping

DOI: 10.4324/9781032664996-10

profession because of personal experiences, and we hope that our narratives allow you space to resonate with our personal connections with
people with disabilities.

Ryan

For most of my career as a psychotherapist, I have worked with able-bodied
and minded clients. However, when I was a young counselor and doctoral
student at the University of North Texas, I had the great privilege of counseling people who were typically low socioeconomic status (SES) at a community counseling clinic, and many were referred by the local mental health
authority. One of my clients whom I counseled for approximately three
years was an adult cisgender male diagnosed with mild IDD and bipolar
disorder. He impacted my professional growth significantly. When I began
working with him, he had recently moved back in with his elderly mother
after living and working independently for several years. He had developed
a dysfunctional relationship with alcohol, lost his job, and could no longer
afford his apartment. His psychiatrist at the local mental health authority, in
my non-medical opinion, had overmedicated him, and he arrived to session
glossy eyed for the first year or so of our work together. My approach with
him was heavily influenced by person-centered work. His goal was to live
and work independently once again. He attained that goal and, as part of
the process, I did some relationship work with him and his mom. As I sit
here writing this sentence, I am thinking about the love, care, and compassion between my client and his mother. I feel a deep sense of teary-eyed joy
as I think about them telling each other how much they will miss seeing
each other every morning, hugging tightly right in front of me. My work
with this client will be with me until my memories fade.

I was faced with examining my own ableism in a brand-new way when
I became a parent of a child with disabilities. My daughter was born with a
rare genetic disorder called Kleefstra syndrome. My wife and I did not know
about her disorder until she was almost 2 years old. Her genetic deletion
resulted in several disabilities and developmental delays, requiring physical
therapy, occupational therapy, and speech therapy. Like many parents of
children with disabilities, we have been on a journey of frustration and disappointment with medical and therapy providers, existential moments of
fear for our daughter's future, and deep joy as we witness her essential self
despite the obstacles her body presents. Along the way, I discovered that
I have the same genetic deletion as my daughter, and subsequently our gen-
eticist established a theory that perhaps my body and mind experienced a far
different gene expressivity outcome. I love my daughter so profoundly and,
as I write this sentence, a figure emerged: a real need and perhaps a lifelong
striving to connect with the way that she sees the world through her eyes,

hears it through her ears, and speaks to it through the unique way that she communicates. When working with clients with disabilities, HST can be a vector for presence, connection, communication, and awareness.

Robin

I can forget I have a learning disability until I must write something professionally. I have a diagnosis of disorder of written expression (DWE) and attention deficit hyperactivity disorder (ADHD). My ADHD is no problem. I drink a lot of coffee and exercise, and I forget I have it. I have more difficulty with DWE. I chose a career in counseling, and professional writing plays a pivotal role in both the path to becoming a counselor and in the practice of professional counseling. Although I would like to describe what it is like to have DWE, I cannot. I do not know how and may never know how. What I do know, however, is how to create a sandtray and tell you about the scene I created. In hopes of providing an educational perspective into DWE, I created a scene (see Figure 8.1) describing what it is like to write this chapter alongside two of my role models, my direct supervisor at work (James) and my LPC-supervisor and former professor (Ryan).

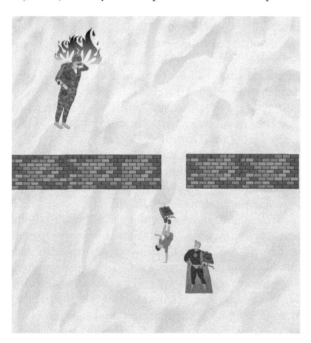

Figure 8.1 Robin's digital sandtray scene. Permission granted by Online Sandtray, Copyright 2024 Dr. Karen Fried.

In my sandtray, my two role models are represented by a superhero and a careless acrobat with books. Both figures are on one side of a brick wall with a large opening. I am on the opposite side of the wall with a pair of binoculars, a book in my hand, and flames over my head. The flames represent my frustration as I wonder how my role models seemed to walk right through the opening in the wall with ease and complete their portions of this chapter. The ideas and concepts I want to contribute are all in my head, but I just do not know how to put them on paper. My work on this chapter has taken countless hours and even more cups of coffee. Despite this, the opportunity to collaborate on this chapter has been worth the challenge, and I hope my efforts may assist those who have the privilege of working with individuals with disabilities.

Mental health and disabilities are something of a family business. My mother is a psychiatric nurse. My father was a family drug and alcohol therapist for 20 years. I rounded things off by becoming a professional counselor. My grandfather was diagnosed with epilepsy. My father has undiagnosed ADHD, Tourette's syndrome, and several learning disabilities. My eldest brother, Andrew, and I share the diagnoses of DWE and ADHD. My brother, Matthew, is diagnosed with dyslexia, Tourette's syndrome, obsessive compulsive disorder (OCD), and ADHD. As a child, my youngest sister, Sophie, was diagnosed with intractable epileptic seizures, and I remember oftentimes hearing the professional prognosis that she would be an invalid for the rest of her life. Thankfully, this prognosis was incorrect. Perhaps the one with the heaviest load to bear, though, is my sister Carley who took on adult-like responsibilities of keeping us organized while finding her own identity and fit in our family system.

I learned a lot from my family that has translated well into my career in counseling. Regarding disabilities, I learned never to use my disability as a crutch, set my own standards, focus on being with people, and have fun. Although my parents always encouraged us never to be ashamed of needing additional resources for learning, it was my grandfather who drove this point home. My grandfather was diagnosed with epilepsy as a child and, as a result, experienced his fair share of trials throughout his life. He was fired from multiple jobs, rejected from serving in the military, and kicked out of college, all due to his seizures. Despite these setbacks, he went on to graduate with a master's degree and started his own small business. Through his life and words, he instilled in me and his other grandchildren the lessons he learned.

Matthew, my brother, exemplified my grandfather's lesson to never use his disabilities as a crutch, and he set his own standards. Matthew was often told it would be a miracle if he graduated from high school, yet he graduated from both high school and college with honors. He describes life with dyslexia as feeling like he must re-learn how to read each time he tries to read anything. Matthew often cites my grandfather and the stories of his perseverance as the motivation to continue striving despite the immense difficulties he faced. Matthew found strength in the knowledge that my grandfather, someone he loved, had faced similar challenges and that my grandfather believed in him.

Although I quickly learned that I could never do all the work for Matthew while we grew up, I also learned that I could stay with him and support him as he worked and studied. Throughout our years of education, Matthew and I would find ourselves in the same class, especially on testing days for homeschool, high school, and community college. On these occasions, I was unable to help Matthew with his work and tests, but I knew that I could stay with him. I would always wait until he had finished his exam and turned it in before I turned in my own test. Matthew shared that he felt more support from my presence with him than from any effort I might have made to do his assignments for him. Looking back, it is apparent how this act of being with someone extends both ways. I now recognize the support I received knowing that someone who struggles as I do also cared about me.

To have fun is another lesson I learned from Matthew. He has always been eager to help me. During my college career, I found Matthew especially helpful with my presentations on life with disabilities. In graduate school, I took a diagnosis class and asked Matthew to help with a presentation to provide insight into the lived experiences of someone with multiple learning disabilities and Tourette's syndrome. Although the presentation received an A, the real reward was observing Matthew shine as a presenter and receive a handshake from the professor.

On another occasion, I was creating a video presentation for an undergraduate class, but Matthew was unavailable to help me with it. Instead of doing the sensible thing and waiting until Matthew was available, I asked my eldest brother, Andrew, if he could depict what Matthew's Tourette's and OCD were like for my recording. Andrew agreed, and the footage was filmed. My professor said this video was the best representation of Tourette's and OCD she had ever seen and asked to continue to use the video for future students. This is a story my family still enjoys telling to this day, and the professor has yet to learn I filmed my other brother. I believe in the power of stories to inspire and, for this reason, I rely heavily on client narratives and Case Studies in this chapter to awaken in you a similar feeling of passion when working with individuals with disabilities.

Both my family background and my personal history with learning disabilities sparked an interest in the limits of striving and human potential when one is faced with issues existing between the psychological and physical. This ultimately provided me with the motivation to pursue a career in counseling. During my graduate program, I sought training in HST. During the training, I began to grasp the power of HST when role play turned into real play and the sandtray I created was processed in real time. The sandtray depicted a scene of guilt and shame associated with serving as my grandfather's caretaker as he approached death while simultaneously wanting to pursue a romantic relationship with the woman who later became my wife. The experience of processing this sandtray fundamentally shaped the approaches I now implement when using a sandtray with clients and dealing with grief, human decency, and the fundamentals of counseling. The trainer, Dr. Steve Armstrong, reflected from both my emotions and my sandtray that I was experiencing intense love for my grandfather as well as grief and loss. He encouraged me to simply tell him about my grandfather, and I have shared this same encouragement with every client dealing with grief and loss.

After processing my sandtray with Steve, he proceeded to make the point that HST, while powerful, does not beat the power of being with clients and "meeting clients where they are." This solidified my understanding of HST as a psychological scalpel that cuts straight to the human soul. My own experience with the sandtray opened my soul to an individual and required that I decide whether to trust this individual. Steve made this an easy decision by meeting me where I was, in my state of love and grief for my grandfather, and being there with me in that experience. This entire experience is best expressed in spiritual terms with the concept of a small, still voice. Steve provided a space in which I could hear the voice of God in my soul by first offering to be a small, still voice himself.

Through this experience, I came to understand HST as a powerful approach that can help clients open up about what is happening inside their souls. Humanistic sandtray therapists gently encourage clients to see what is there and to see that they are not alone. Some clients experience this latter point in a spiritual sense, whereas others experience it differently with the knowledge that I, as a therapist, am with them. Regardless, HST provides a space for clients to know they are not alone in that moment and in their experiencing. It was this knowledge of not being alone that enacted significant change in my life, brought resolution to an issue I was facing at the time, and fostered my desire to work with individuals from an HST approach. I wanted to use HST to see if individuals impacted significantly by mental health diagnoses could benefit.

Upon graduating from my graduate program, I accepted a position with a local mental health agency where I provide trauma therapy to people with disabilities, particularly those diagnosed with IDD. I have had the privilege of sitting with clients who are diagnosed with IDD as they become immersed in deeply symbolic scenes. One example that comes to mind is a scene in which a lost princess finds acceptance in becoming one of the forest creatures. A second example is the memory of a client gazing proudly at a sandtray full of people miniatures. The client explained that each miniature represented a different aspect of his personality, and he finally gained a sense of self-understanding.

James

My wife and I moved to Fort Worth from East Texas to raise our boys in an exciting city with zoos and water parks. I got a job at the local mental health authority in Tarrant County and worked as a manager and counselor. I got a great opportunity to transfer to a division of the agency that provided services to children and adults diagnosed with IDD. My focus coming into this new position was to figure out ways to bring psychotherapy to this population. I had a general idea it would be a challenge counseling them, because I worked previously as a residential trainer at a group home for adults with IDD right out of college. I was familiar with their cognitive and verbal limitations.

One of the elements of psychotherapy on which therapists come to rely is the conversational flow of sessions. Whether a therapist employs psychodynamic therapy, family systems work, cognitive behavior therapy, dialectical behavior therapy, eye movement desensitization reprocessing, motivational interviewing, sandtray, reality therapy, person-centered therapy, or internal family system therapy, all these approaches rely on the ability of clients to express their feelings and communicate verbally. I have always been anchored in person-centered therapy. For me, Carl Rogers' understanding of the powerful healing nature of the therapeutic relationship resonated to my core. So, in trying to figure out how to work with the IDD population, I went back to my roots in person-centered therapy. I have practiced child-centered play therapy, too, so I felt armed with a relevant approach for working with the IDD population.

I wanted to find a way to work with adults with IDD without treating them as children. I wanted to meet them where they were at. I wanted to create an environment of respect, kindness, trust, and authenticity. I realized quickly when I started working with individuals diagnosed with various developmental disabilities like down syndrome, ASD, fetal alcohol syndrome, and IDD that their ability to express their feelings verbally was limited. They suffered from the same painful emotions all humans face, yet they often lacked the language to describe their inner worlds.

I first used motivational interviewing, because it has elements of person-centered therapy and focused on learning what clients want and how to help them achieve their goals. The first challenge I ran into with using this

approach is that my clients with IDD are often "people pleasers" in counseling. They often tell me what they think I want to hear. Sometimes, they
are desperate for a friendship. Initially, they may seem interested in learning
counseling self-care techniques but, in my experience, my clients genuinely
want a friend who cares and listens. So, I realized that all the counseling
theories I spent the last 20 years learning and desperately wanted this population to have access to would have to be adapted in a way to overcome
the people-pleasing dynamic that I so commonly experienced with them in
counseling.

Subsequently, I concluded that I was discriminating in working with this
population because I was creating assumptions that were false. The people-
pleasing dynamic in therapy can occur with any client. Commonly referred
to as transference, this is when clients project their dreams, wishes, needs,
preferences, and desires into the counseling relationship. When I realized
how transference was presented within my therapeutic relationships, I had
an "aha" moment that hit me like a ton of bricks. This population is not
challenging to engage with in counseling; they are more transparent and
authentic than non-IDD populations with whom I had worked. I had few
colleagues to talk about this realization with back then because I did not
know many counselors working with IDD.

My exposure to co-morbid mental health diagnoses and IDD brought
me into contact with Harvey's (2012) work with trauma-informed care.
Harvey stated that systems of care often mandate behavior support services when clients diagnosed with IDD demonstrate challenging behaviors. Behavior support services usually include a plan that is developed to
help caregivers learn ways to support the individual to reduce challenging
behaviors. Harvey advocated for counseling services for people with IDD
in tandem with a behavior support plan that attends to their challenging
behaviors. I started using sandtray as a trauma-informed approach with
individuals diagnosed with IDD. Sandtray therapy provided a new platform
for my clients to express themselves. My clients could access their emotions through animals, rocks, trees, people, houses, fences, religious figures,
fantasy figures, and so much more. I was unsure if it would work in the
beginning, but I witnessed a few sandtray scenes that ignited my passion
even more.

Addressing Ableism in HST

Just as humanistic sandtray therapists are tasked to engage in reflective practice in terms of their clients' racial, ethnic, spiritual or religious, gender,
sexual, socioeconomic, and indigenous identities (see Chapter 6), we find
it imperative that they examine their ableism and its relationship to the

therapeutic process with clients with disabilities. This inner exploration may lead you to discover the ways in which your ableism presents itself in your therapeutic approach and even your office. For example, I (Ryan) used to practice in an intensive outpatient program. The office was in a business park on the second floor. However, there was no elevator to the second floor—only a set of long, narrow stairs. I did not think much of this as an obstacle other than my own breathless arrival to our practice space a few times a week. I was faced with the collective ableism of myself and the group of practitioners with whom I worked when I ran an HST training and one of the practitioners who attended the training walked with the assistance of crutches due to her cerebral palsy. She was able to climb the stairs, yet I wondered what I was thinking when I offered the training there. It is an image in my mind that I will never forget. Later in this chapter, we will discuss how to create a non-ableist physical space in your consultation room.

According to Sevcik et al. (2022), one of the ableist myths of working with adults with severe disabilities is that they "only have simple thoughts, feelings, understandings, and needs" (p. 420). Sevcik et al. noted that often these individuals are denied "opportunities to engage more fully in rich conversations" (p. 420). They described their interview with a parent of a man who was congenitally deafblind, read braille at a first-grade level, and fully comprehended adult literature on audiobook. It is a good example of the complexities involved with severe disabilities and the false assumptions that practitioners might create regarding a clients' limitations without evidence. Sevcik et al. challenged practitioners to avoid basing their evaluation of a client's capacities solely on expressive communication abilities or even on one modality of receptive communication. Therefore, a humanistic sandtray therapist should never assume that a client who has disabilities is unsuitable for one mode of therapy, such as HST, based on the therapist's perception of an isolated communication ability. We believe in the power of exploration and discovery, and if your clients with disabilities demonstrate openness to sandtray, we encourage you to trust their perceptions.

Case Study 8.1: Cheryl

Cheryl is a 33-year-old single mother. Over the course of treatment, she went from being homeless to being a full-time employee living in her own home with custody of her 7-year-old son. When she and I (Robin) started working together, Cheryl had moved back in with her parents and regained custody of her son. There were two consistent themes from Cheryl's HST work: the presence of her son in each of her sandtray scenes and the strength and meaning she gained from being a mother. It was common for Cheryl to bring her son with her to our sessions. On one occasion, Cheryl and her son each created a sandtray and explained their trays to one another. Cheryl used an opera mask to express how she often puts on a mask of happiness and that she does experience sadness, even though she may not show it. Cheryl said it was important that her son knows that it is never because of him that her sadness occurs. Cheryl's son expressed gratitude for his mom's description and explained how the sandtray and the mask figurine helped him understand what his mom was sharing. On his side of the sandtray, Cheryl's son shared how spending time with his mom doing mundane tasks and chores brought him intense joy and happiness. He expressed worry that she tries too hard to provide him with toys when all he wants is to spend time with her. By participating in HST, both mother and son gained the awareness that they each provide joy and meaning to one another.

Wisdom Versus Intelligence

Kaufman (2013) argued that there is little to no correlation between intellectual functioning and wisdom or intellectual functioning and creativity. We have seen this reality manifested in work with clients who have IQs in the mid-50s to 70s. These clients routinely demonstrate areas of insight and wisdom when creating and processing a sandtray and have little-to-no difficulty making use of the HST approach. Following are Case Studies that demonstrate the kind of deep-seated wisdom that clients with IDD have demonstrated through HST with us.

Case Study 8.2: Alesha

Alesha is a 27-year-old female living in a group home, dealing with issues of anger and rejection. When working on processing the conflictual relationship with her stepmother, Alesha asked if she could divide the sandtray in half. On one side, she placed figures representing happiness and joy. On the other side, she placed figures representing the repressed anger and rejection associated with her stepmother. In sharing her thought process behind splitting the sandtray in half, Alesha explained how she thought it would be easier to process the difficult memories if she also thought of pleasant memories and things she enjoyed. In this explanation, Alesha described the eye movement desensitization and reprocessing (EMDR) technique of laying down tracks as part of the accelerated information processing model, a technique that bridges traumatic memories that are maladaptively stored with pleasant and processed memories that are stored adaptively (Shapiro, 2017).

Case Study 8.3: Chris

Chris is an 18-year-old male living at home and dealing with intense social anxiety, isolation, and identity issues. Through HST, Chris demonstrated insight into his psychosocial development. Chris created a scene in which he was stuck in the middle of a triangular desert. At each point of the triangle was a figure representing a different facet of his life: friendship, Jewish faith, and high school. In processing the scene, Chris shared the uncertainty he felt about not knowing in which direction to go and the anxiety that was directing him to explore each point on the triangle. Ultimately, Chris felt fearful of what he might leave behind in choosing any one point of the triangle above the other two. In this session, Chris depicted the identity vs. role confusion stage of psychological development during which individuals engage in the exploration of and commitment to the areas of ideology, vocation, and relationship (Marcia, 1993). Additionally, the anxiety directing Chris to explore each point of his ideology, vocation, and relationship triangle seems to have helped him avoid fear of exploration, which is a common pitfall resulting in identity foreclosure.

Case Study 8.4: Eric

Eric is a 44-year-old male living with his sister and attending a work program where he packages supplies for a local food bank. Eric is processing the complex grief and trauma associated with the death of his abusive father. When working with Eric, I (Robin) am often confronted with the limitations of my portable sandtray figures. According to Eric, my collection lacks "Power Rangers to feel powerful" and a dog figurine that is an accurate representation of his dog, Gadget. Eric is a resourceful, natural leader, and he finds ways to make my limited selection of figures work for his needs. On one occasion, Eric was using the sandtray to describe a difficult memory of life when he lived with his father. For Eric, it was important to depict the positive memories of time spent with his father, like the time they took their dogs for a walk, despite the abusive relationship. In creating this scene, Eric pointed out that I did not have a dog leash figurine. Although I apologized and assured him that I would try to find a leash figurine for our future sessions, Eric stated, without hesitation, that "we could just make one right now." He then proceeded to make a dog leash out of a piece of yarn.

Intersection of Disability and Trauma

One of our guiding principles when working with individuals with traumatic backgrounds is inspired by John Green's (2013) book *The Fault in Our Stars*: the problem with pain is that it demands to be felt and is not easily ignored. C. S. Lewis (2001) came to a similar conclusion earlier when discussing pain's insistence on being attended to and the inability to ignore emotional and physical pain. When applied to HST, these ideas can alleviate the pressure a therapist might feel to address traumatic issues which they know exist but that the client does not readily see or bring up on their own. By definition, trauma means wound, and anyone who has had a wound can understand that it comes with pain. Put plainly, pain demands to be felt, and it will make itself known during HST.

Case Study 8.5: Gustavo

Gustavo was a Latino cisgender male in his early fifties diagnosed with IDD and bipolar disorder who was living in a group home. I (James) began seeing him because he engaged often in non-suicidal self-injury (NSSI), cutting himself with whatever he could find. He would break glass windows and then cut his arm. He would find soda cans in the street and cut the bottoms of his feet. He had been performing NSSI since he was 13 years old. His vocabulary was limited, but he could hold short conversations and would continue talking if verbally guided. He and his sister were sexually molested by his grandfather when they were young. His parents were violent and went to jail frequently. He saw his father have a heart attack one Saturday morning and die on the kitchen table right in front of his eyes. What family he had left placed him in a group home when he was in his twenties. He liked talking about country music and listening to songs on YouTube. He liked the old country singers that I liked such as George Jones, Conway Twitty, Hank Williams, and Waylon Jennings. He would get so excited talking about fishing. He had lots of memories of fishing, and some were complex, because his grandfather molested him when they would go on fishing trips.

I started prompting him to use the sand tray. He started building scenes with ease and comfort. He seemed thoughtful about where he wanted to place figures. During one sandtray session, he grabbed a handful of sharks, snakes, and dangerous sea creatures and placed them throughout the sand. He then placed an old handsome blonde adventurous person right in the middle of the creatures. He described it as he was building the scene, "he is getting eaten," "he is bleeding in the ocean and the fish are taking small bites of him," "there is blood all around."

When he left the session, as I was cleaning the sand tray, I got a felt sense of what he was trying to communicate through his sandtray scene. The sharks biting this guy are just like my client cutting himself. The small bites of the floating man were like the small cuts he would give himself. The man was also floating in the ocean and getting eaten. My client probably felt like that all the time as a kid, and these feelings emerged for him as he created his tray: lonely, scared, terrorized, and abandoned. When he cut, the feelings shifted to his body. He could control the pain in his body, but not the mental and emotional pain.

Over time, his sandtray scenes told the story of his life. His trays displayed worlds in which he wished he lived. Over time his trays reflected hope. His common trays were of a penguin fishing off a bridge with all kinds of animals drinking from a creek's stream below. Penguins have learned how to survive in cold places. He shared feelings of shame, ridicule, loneliness, fear, sadness, and longing. He missed his grandfather, and he loved him dearly. His favorite memories were with his grandfather.

Working with him taught me (James) how complex we humans can be. Our work together taught me the value of sandtray when counseling clients who have a painful history of trauma. Working with Gustavo in the sand was a transformative experience between us as therapist and client.

People with IDD are incredibly vulnerable to trauma (Presnell, Keesler, & Thomas-Giyer, 2022), with estimates of likelihood for abuse or neglect ranging from three to six times more than the general population (Hulbert-Williams et al., 2013). Scotti et al. (2012) reported that more than 70 percent of people with IDD had at least one traumatic event. Prevalence rates of post-traumatic stress in the IDD population reportedly are 10 percent to 40 percent (Daveny et al., 2019; Mevissen et al., 2020; Nieuwenhuis et al., 2019). Our clients' stories of being marginalized and forgotten are all too common among those with disabilities. Their feelings and experiences are often labeled as "challenging behaviors," which are overshadowed by their diagnosis, and the result is that their trauma stories often go untold. The way that systems of care operate can bring up clients' associations with traumatic experiences, too. Some of our clients have expressed to us that they believed we were "writing them up" when we would take behavioral notes in counseling. These data sheets, as they are often called, are pulled out in front of clients while staff quickly write up the antecedent events to behavior incidents. Getting "written up" often leads us to learning about clients' feelings of shame, frustration, and worry that they are "getting in trouble."

We consider HST a trauma-informed approach and, therefore, believe that sandtray therapy can provide a safe space for clients with disabilities to explore their trauma experiences. Herman (2022) expressed the importance of connection and establishing a safe environment with people recovering from trauma. Moreover, Harvey (2012) advocated for practitioners to facilitate trauma-informed approaches with clients who have disabilities. In our experiences, establishing a safe and trusting relationship can be a challenge working with clients diagnosed with IDD because so many of them have emerged out of trauma and may live in chronically stressful environments. Their external worlds are often tightly controlled. They are often told what to do and where to go. They are told what to wear and what to eat, or they are left alone to the endless supplies of video games and Internet entertainment. Therefore, our clients have often expected us to be another in a long line of people controlling their lives; however, when therapy is consistent, and caregivers support the therapeutic process to unfold, then the outcomes can be measured in many more ways than simply "reduced challenging behaviors." In our sandtray work with this population, we have witnessed outcomes like freedom of expression, improved self-esteem, emotional self-regulation, discovered strengths, and stronger connections with family, friends, and caregivers.

In our experiences, there can be a dilemma in knowing the detailed trauma history of a client diagnosed with IDD or related disabilities and having been trained in evidence-based approaches to treating trauma. As a clinician, it can be tempting to use the knowledge and insight obtained from the caregivers of clients to inform a directive approach to therapy. The Center for

Substance Abuse Treatment (2014), however, cautions against the risk of re-traumatization when traumatic issues are brought up with clients before they have adequate supports. With the development of evidence-based, trauma-informed approaches like EMDR (Shapiro, 2017), it is easy for therapists to think that they are withholding necessary treatment from clients who are disabled by choosing not to bring up a client's traumatic history if the client fails to do so themselves. If you are a trained trauma therapist, it can be tempting to encourage a client to create sandtray scenes about specific traumatic events and to draw connections for clients. It can be a challenge, regardless of your therapeutic approach, to resist this temptation to bring up a traumatic past with a good intention toward client healing.

Case Study 8.6: Ian

Ian is a 15-year-old male living with his grandmother. His biological mother died by suicide. This specific session with Ian provides a lighthearted example of how a client can respond to feeling pressured to address a traumatic issue prematurely. When asked to create a scene describing his biological mother, Ian created a detailed scene describing the canned ravioli he made for his sister the previous evening. Logically, I (Robin) questioned Ian on his understanding of the sandtray prompt. Ian informed me that although he did understand the original sandtray prompt, he does not answer "pesky questions from nosey counselors."

A unique difference between HST and other more directive trauma-informed approaches is the non-directive nature of HST. This ultimately allows for the principle of "pain demanding to be felt" to be applied. Ultimately, the sandtray allows humanistic sandtray therapists to bypass these dilemmas by encouraging clients to create the scenes they want to create. Often, clients will create scenes that describe pain and trauma without prompting from therapists and will include pain and trauma that was not discovered during their initial assessments or intake processes.

Case Study 8.7: Mike

Mike is a 23-year-old single male living at home. Mike has an exten-sive history of physical trauma resulting from violence by individ-uals he met over the Internet. Mike's mother is his medical power of attorney, and she assisted in completing Mike's initial assessment. Due to conflicting schedules, Mike and his mother worked to complete the initial assessment and intake individually. In reviewing this information, each party presented a significantly different history of trauma. Mike's mother emphasized the physical abuse and mistreatment from individuals online. Mike emphasized the medical trauma resulting from his many physical and medical disabilities. Both Mike and his mother provided detailed accounts of traumatic history that had potential to benefit from a more directive approach. However, I (Robin) decided to take a non-directive approach in working with Mike and encouraged him to create sandtray scenes focused more on rapport building than traumatic history.

While processing a scene about his favorite memories, Mike began to describe an embarrassing memory that was more directly linked to issues of trust and relationships. As Mike shared this embarrassing memory, what ultimately came up was another memory of being the perpetrator of sexual molestation as a child. This memory ultimately led to a discussion of Mike's lifetime struggle with survivor's guilt related to his twin. The session concluded with Mike developing an increased awareness of how he overcompensates for his traumatic past with hypersexuality and physical aggression. It is interesting to note that none of the issues addressed during this session had been noted in the client's initial assessment. It is possible that all of this could have been missed had we focused on specific traumatic memories instead of rapport building and that Mike would have closed up or been re-traumatized.

Practical Adaptations to and Inclusion in HST

In this section, we will discuss some practical considerations in using HST with clients with disabilities, which is based on the notion of *disability inclusion*. Disability inclusion "allows for people with disabilities to take advantage of the benefits of the same health promotion and prevention activities experienced by people who do not have a disability" (Centers for Disease Control and Prevention, 2020, para. 4). In your HST practice, we encourage you to note ways in which you can align with disability inclusion practices that reflect concepts of the social model of disability. Humanistic sandtray therapists actively seek ways to remove barriers to clients' access to sandtray therapy. First, we will discuss guidance on having an inclusive collection of miniatures. Then, we will discuss adaptations pursuant to two kinds of disabilities: neurodivergence and physical disabilities, with the caveat that you may have clients who have multiple disabilities across both categories.

Miniatures

As with other populations presented in this book, we recommend that you actively build your sandtray collection to include miniatures that have potential to capture symbols and experiences common to people with disabilities. Following is a non-exhaustive list to consider:

- *People with various disabilities:* Collection of people with various seen disabilities (e.g., adult and child in wheelchair or crutches). Attend to intersectional identities when using people miniatures.
- *Objects used in various therapy and medical environments:* A tablet could represent augmented and alternative communication (AAC) hardware, swings and blocks could represent occupational and physical therapy paraphernalia, medical devices, tools, and equipment including plastic tubes, physician and nurse miniatures.
- *Body parts:* Internal organs, severed limbs, digits (e.g., fingers), eyeballs, ears, tongue, and nose.
- *Trauma symbols:* People physically abusing others, self-injurious miniature, jail cell, handcuffs, and a mummy.
- *Empowerment, hope, and freedom symbols:* Pegasus, raised fist, butterflies, rainbow, treasure chest, coins and dollar bills, and the Statue of Liberty.

Neurodivergence and Humanistic Sandtray Therapy

Early in its history, Buhler (1951) established sandtray as an assessment tool using her World Test for children with developmental ability differences. In addition, Tanguay (2009) reported on her adaptation of the World Test for adults with developmental ability differences. Smith (2012) described a practical model of using sandplay with children in special education settings. Our review of literature revealed that sandplay seems to be the dominant sand therapy approach to working with people who are neurodivergent. However, Komarek (2020) implemented Homeyer and Sweeney's (2023) cross-theoretical approach to sandtray with adults diagnosed with IDD and co-morbid mental health diagnoses. She found that sandtray had a meaningful impact on participants' psychological distress and well-being. Caregivers also reported positive changes in emotional expression and interpersonal relationships.

We propose that HST is well suited for clients who are neurodivergent, which includes clients who are diagnosed with down syndrome, ASD, and IDD, among many others. The HST emphasis on the therapeutic relationship and its exploratory stance provide a therapeutic experience that is focused on acceptance, experiencing, and openness. In HST, practitioners avoid focusing on behavioral change or management and have no predetermined expectations of their clients. However, we encourage you to consider potential modifications to your HST practice with neurodivergent clients. Following are distinct ways that you can adapt HST to work with clients with neurodivergent-related disabilities: establish contact with caregivers and the client's system of care; provide options to replace sand in the tray; and adapt to clients' expressive and receptive communication processes and abilities.

To *establish contact with caregivers and the client's system of care*, we recommend creating an effective professional relationship with the important people, including professionals, in your client's life. For example, neurodivergent clients may have other kinds of therapists assisting them with their development, such as speech, occupational, and physical therapists. Even if you are an outside practitioner, securing a release of information to work alongside other professionals and caregivers may be of great benefit for your client's overall functioning. By caregivers, we mean parents and potentially group home managers. However, to be clear, you should always operate with the same healthy boundaries as you would any other client. Humanistic sandtray therapists operate from an ethical and clinical prerogative of what is best for the client *according to the client*.

Providing options to replace sand in the tray is a response we recommend for neurodivergent clients who may have sensitivity to the feeling of sand. Therefore, you may want to have a second sand tray in which you can use dry rice, beans, or even marbles as the "sand." Kinetic sand may be another option as it has a different feel to it from regular sand. Work with your client by providing samples to establish what kind of medium might be an acceptable replacement.

Adapting to clients' expressive and receptive communication processes and abilities involves gathering information about how they typically communicate to others, receive and comprehend information from others, and in what ways you can modify your therapeutic process given these data. We recommend that you gather established assessment data from their care team, if they have one, as well as from parents and the client themselves. If your client uses an AAC device, explore with them its use during sandtray. We certainly would not use HST until we know a client's communication abilities and methods.

Case Study 8.8: Walter

I (James) worked with a young adolescent male, Walter, who was diagnosed with IDD and who had lost his leg in a gunshot accident. He was a quiet and reserved young man and limited in verbal conversation. The typical small talk at the beginning of therapy was not working, and I was losing his attention. I pulled out all the sandtray miniatures and a small sand tray and asked him to create a world of anything he wanted. He immediately went to work organizing the figures and building up the sand to the levels he wanted. He created an elaborate scene of a zoo with all kinds of animals behind fences. One of the animals was a gorilla behind closed quarters. He placed people outside the fence and described them as throwing things at the gorilla and laughing at the gorilla. This sandtray scene opened the door for him to express how he felt when other kids at school laughed at him and made fun of his missing leg. This sandtray world felt sad and discouraging. It depicted his pain, suffering, and isolation and he made it all come alive with some of the most visceral images I had seen in sandtray at this point in my career.

When working with clients who have limited verbal abilities, creating a sandtray scene provides them with a medium to express what they are experiencing and what feelings may be locked away. The sandtray provided an opportunity to process his feelings and experiences, and the world he created was safely contained in the tray along with the unconditional positive regard from the therapeutic relationship. He became more verbal in therapy and his confidence in himself and his ability to express himself became increasingly apparent. Initially, his sandtray world on the surface appeared to reflect the trauma and aftermath of losing his leg, yet there were other hidden meanings that emerged. His experiences of struggling with cognitive and intellectual delays and how his peers treated him revealed much deeper complex trauma. Unfortunately, such is the case often in working with individuals diagnosed with IDD.

When adapting HST to individuals diagnosed with IDD, we have found success in starting with concrete prompts during initial sessions and then incorporating more open-ended prompts as the therapeutic relationship develops. This method allows clients both the time needed to become comfortable with the sandtray and to tap into their imagination and creativity. The progression from concrete prompts to open-ended prompts is meant to prevent a client from feeling overwhelmed. We have found that clients diagnosed with IDD have people-pleasing tendencies often that manifest during initial sessions, especially in instances where they are unable to make use of the sandtray. Clients can become overwhelmed when a desire to please the therapist coexists with an open-ended sandtray prompt that they do not understand.

Case Study 8.9: Brandon

Brandon is a 26-year-old male living with his mother. He is dealing with trauma from authority figures in high school, anger outbursts, and a feeling of being easily overwhelmed when faced with adversity. In an early session, I (Robin) encouraged Brandon to create a scene describing his world. Brandon thought about the prompt for a minute and declined the request to create that scene. Instead, he requested I stick with the basics such as talking, listening, and sharing information about human development. Three months into our therapeutic relationship, Brandon shared that he was embarrassed when I asked him, in that early session, to create the scene describing his world. Brandon wanted to engage in the HST approach I suggested, but he was confused by the prompt and what I was asking him to do with the sandtray. Upon learning this, we collaborated on a prompt to create a scene where the figures describe his friends. With this prompt, Brandon created a scene full of concrete symbolism in which he used pyramids and a sphinx figure to represent friends in Egypt and a police figure to represent the friends he has on the police force.

In addition, humanistic sandtray therapists can use sandtray to help clients *practice* effective communication. Case Study 8.1 reinforces this concept. In this case study, a mother and child both use the sandtray to communicate more effectively with one another and develop their relationship. Cheryl's son created a sandtray that gave him insight into his desire to spend more time with his mother. Subsequently, he used the scene he had created and processed as a reference when communicating to his father a desire to spend more time with his mother. The sandtray provided a common language each of them could use to express their inner thoughts and desires to the other.

With adaptations, HST can provide benefits like those of many classic therapeutic techniques including the client writing a letter about their thoughts, needs, boundaries, and wishes and reading this letter to family members. HST can make a client's ideas, thoughts, and feelings more accessible, and clients can take pictures of their trays to use for reference in communication going forward. In our experiences, it is helpful to introduce the sandtray early on and to carefully gauge the client's reactions to determine your next steps. If the client expresses interest in the HST approach, proceed with concrete sandtray prompts that will build rapport. However, if the client is hesitant about the HST approach, wait and re-introduce the tray again after issues and themes have been identified. We strongly recommend that you follow your client's lead.

Acting Out Versus Creating Then Processing a Sandtray

Several of our clients have adapted the sandtray on their own and without prompting. They have used the sandtray in a non-traditional manner by acting out scenes in the tray and merging the creation and processing phases of HST. For clients who have developmental disabilities, the traditional HST approach in which clients first create a scene in the sandtray in silence and then progress into the processing phase where they describe the scene can be challenging. We have found that some clients need to combine the creation and processing phases. When asked to separate these phases, some clients can become confused and dysregulated.

Case Study 8.10: John

John is a 13-year-old male living with his father. We engaged in HST each week, and he consistently blended the creation and processing phases. In our initial session, I (Robin) encouraged John to first create a scene and then to tell me about the scene. John would become dysregulated and implement self-soothing behaviors when I set limits requiring him to separate the HST process into its two distinct parts of creation and processing. Over time, I found that John benefited most from the use of reflections of feelings and meaning while simultaneously creating and processing a sandtray prompt.

Case Study 8.11: Greg

Greg is a 44-year-old male living with his sister and attending a work program where he packages supplies for a local food bank. In one session, Greg was using the sandtray to process a breakup with his girlfriend. I (Robin) had encouraged Greg to first create the scene and then process the scene, but Greg found it challenging to use the sandtray in this manner because he could not remember what each figure represented. We decided to try the same prompt a second time with Greg using the sandtray in a way that felt natural to him. He, too, ended up combining the creation and processing phases of HST. In his second attempt, Greg flawlessly described the pain and hurt he was experiencing from his breakup as he created the scene itself. Greg remembered which character represented himself, his friends, his ex-girlfriend, and her new boyfriend. It is noteworthy that this breakup and the emotions associated with it were prevalent topics across several sessions. Greg ultimately found a new girlfriend and created a sandtray scene in which he became friends with his ex-girlfriend and celebrated the happiness she found in her new relationship.

Polarities

Polarities work can take place with clients diagnosed with disabilities and may need alteration to respond to their developmental abilities. One polarity that appears in client trays relates to their life as it is now versus their life struggle-free. We find that individuals in the concrete and formal operations stages of cognitive development find it difficult to articulate verbally their current life situation—as well as a world in which their problems are resolved. HST plays a pivotal role in making this polarity more accessible to clients by making it more concrete. First, the therapist can encourage the client to create a scene describing their current world, theme, or issue on one side of the tray using figures that are relevant to the therapeutic topic. In this way, the therapist provides a concrete application of one half of the client's polarity. Next, the therapist can encourage the client to use the other half of the tray to create a scene in which their issue no longer exists. The therapist can explain that in this half of the sandtray, the problem at hand has been resolved, and the scene here is of a world in which their struggles are no longer around. For example, I (Robin) worked with a client in which we integrated her polarity of her current struggles versus a future in which she has none into a sandtray prompt; she created a world in which her stepmother no longer existed. Over the next several sessions, the client experimented with completely removing the stepmother figure from the tray and interacting with the stepmother figure directly. The results of this process can vary based on the client, but these steps allow for the benefits of processing a common polarity in HST.

Case Study 8.12: Simon

Simon is a 46-year-old male living in a group home. He has been dealing with addiction and trauma from the day he discovered his father
dead. Following a sandtray prompt based on his polarity of his current struggle versus a problem-free future, Simon created the life he
wanted on one side of the sandtray and the life he is currently living
on the other side of the sandtray. Through this exercise with a more
concrete polarity, Simon was able to identify the goal of finding an
intimate partner. The real benefit, though, was the sense of gratitude
Simon felt upon noticing the similarities that existed on both sides of
the tray. Simon identified friendship, a home, a source of income, and
access to food and transportation as facets of both the life he wanted
and the life he is currently living.

In addition, HST can benefit clients with various developmental disabilities
in exploring polarities as intrapsychic parts.

Case Study 8.13: Cheryl Revisited

During a session with Cheryl, I (Robin) encouraged her to create a
sandtray scene describing her inner child. Cheryl chose miniatures to
represent her current-day self as she observed three versions of her
inner child. The first inner child miniature was molested as a young
girl. The second inner child miniature was the teenager subjected to
domestic violence. The third inner child miniature was the reckless
20-year-old engaging in promiscuous sexual activity. I encouraged
Cheryl to interact with any or all of these inner child figures, and
she did. Cheryl shared how all three inner child miniatures shared a
common theme of needing to be told by her current-day self that the
traumatic events of her past were not their fault.

Physical and Mobility Disabilities and Humanistic Sandtray Therapy

Physical disabilities include a wide range of functionality and causes. People
with acquired disabilities may have one or more amputated body parts,
paralysis, or a medical condition that causes them to need assistance with

gross or fine motor abilities. There are other physical disabilities that are genetic in nature, such as cerebral palsy, missing or differently shaped limbs, or developmental coordination disorder. Clients with physical or mobility disabilities may also have a diagnosis related to neurodivergent disabilities. There are two fundamental ways that humanistic sandtray therapists can engage in an anti-ableist and inclusive sandtray process: providing equitable physical access to the sandtray space and collection, and potential assistance in creating the sandtray scene itself.

Humanistic sandtray therapists can *provide equitable physical access to the sandtray space and collection* in multiple ways. First, the office space itself should be accessible—think of my (Ryan's) experience working on the second floor of a building with no elevator. Second, arrange your office so that it can accommodate the clearance necessary for people who use wheelchairs or similar mobility assistance to be able to enter, navigate around your office to access your sandtray collection, and exit your office safely and without physical obstacles. We recommend you review the 2010 Americans with Disability Act standards for specific guidance (U.S. Department of Justice Civil Rights Division, 2010).

Now let us talk about *potential assistance in creating the sandtray scene.* If you have a client who is a good fit for and who is interested in sandtray therapy, and the nature of that client's physical disability is such that moving miniatures in the ways that they wish requires assistance, then we recommend that you first have a discussion with the client regarding how they envision your role. *Never assume a client needs help.* If they request assistance from you to create their scene, never assume *how* they want your help. Ask them directly how they want you to help. Do they want you to pick the objects up for them and bring them over to the tray? Do they want you to set up the scene under their direction? Perhaps they are unsure—invite them to try it out, and it may be that you both discover invalid assumptions about their abilities to physically pick up the miniatures and create the scene of their choosing. Your client might be able to select the miniatures they want but their fine motor abilities limit autonomous movement to place the miniatures in the scene the way they want them. The intersection of their physical disabilities and creation of the scene can be nuanced; however, it can be a meaningful process and ultimately is an effort to respect the client's autonomy.

For example, one of us (Robin) once worked with a client who was primarily wheelchair bound. During session, she requested help in gathering figures from the shelves and placing them in the sand tray. My initial thought was to reply with a child-centered play therapy (CCPT) returning responsibility statement. Thankfully, my Southern manners ruled out, and I proceeded to pick up figures at her recommendation and put them into the sand tray instead. Subsequently, the client was able to arrange the figures within the tray and enter the processing phase of HST. Helping this client with the creation of her sandtray ultimately enhanced her progress in treatment by allowing for immediacy as I asked her what it was like to receive help. This experience led to a touching moment in which the client, through tears, was able to express gratitude for the woman who had been her physical aid for several years. Additionally, this client processed her feelings of guilt stemming from a recent physical therapy appointment in which she used her physical disability as a crutch to avoid participating in the exercises.

Using HST in In-Home and Group Home Settings

Larson et al. (2017) reported that through 2015, approximately 1.46 million people diagnosed with IDD received services from state agencies. Of those people, 5 percent lived in a host or foster family home, 26 percent lived in a group home, and 58 percent lived in a family member's home. Due to associated environmental barriers such as access to transportation and poverty, many clients with disabilities, particularly clients who are diagnosed with IDD, receive therapeutic services in their homes or in group home settings. Two of us (Robin and James) currently work for the disabilities division of a local mental health authority, and the foremost setting in which we conduct sandtray therapy with older child, adolescent, and adult clients diagnosed with IDD is at their residences, typically in-home where they live with family or in a group home. We have developed multiple recommendations for humanistic sandtray therapists when providing therapy in these settings.

Benefits

There are benefits to using HST during an in-home session, both at an individual residence and a group home. The in-home setting provides the therapist with opportunities to take a detailed look into the client's daily life and world and can allow for a deeper empathic connection. Access to care for the client is readily available in-home, and there is typically an opportunity for the immediate application of awareness gained from processing a sandtray, particularly when associated with the client's space or relationships at home.

Case Study 8.14: Kendall

Kendall is a 44-year-old male living in a group home. He is working on issues of trust, belonging, and autonomy after being moved from group home to group home. Kendall is having trouble maintaining steady employment, and his truck was repossessed, which made it impossible for him to go for a drive. While working with the sandtray, Kendall experienced a new perspective that the group home manager's decision to decline Kendall's request to drive her car was not a rejection of Kendall as a person or an indicator of the group home manager's lack of trust in him. Later in the session, the group home manager walked by. Kendall flagged her down to double check his new interpretation of her behavior and expressed significant relief when his group home manager confirmed that she did not think he was a bad person who was unworthy of trust.

Considerations

Despite these benefits, there are several considerations when using HST during in-home sessions. These include issues with portability, confidentiality, and depth of processing. We will discuss each issue and offer Case Studies to highlight how we have managed them.

Portability

When working as a traveling therapist and seeing clients in-home, considerations arise regarding physical space. Sessions that are in-home sessions or in another community setting typically have less physical space available for people and objects when compared with an office setting. As a result, the sand tray may need to be smaller in size and easily transportable. The number of miniatures included in a portable sandtray kit may also need to be condensed.

Oftentimes, in-home sessions take place in common areas with a table and chairs like the living room, dining room, or kitchen. Although a table provides a place to set up the portable sand tray and miniatures, it can block the therapist's view of the client and their body language. Therefore, it can be beneficial for both the therapist and client to sit on the same side of the table or for the therapist and client to each sit on a different side of the same table corner. This allows the therapist to observe the client more effectively and gives the opportunity to notice behaviors like the tapping of feet, the crossing of legs, or the fidgeting of hands, which can indicate that the client is becoming overwhelmed. For example, one of my (Robin's) clients in a group home became closed often when discussing issues in session and required my aid in tapping on her knees, similar to bilateral stimulation in EMDR, to process difficult themes during HST. Sitting on the same side of the table as the client made it easier to assist the client when needed.

Moreover, the space in which a therapy session takes place can impact the client's willingness to explore deeper issues. In our experiences, a lack of privacy or the occurrence of frequent interruptions by other members of the household during session has caused clients to be less willing to go in-depth on issues. A client's willingness to explore deeper issues can also be impacted by the physical size of a sand tray and the quantity of miniatures available to them. When working with clients in-home, it is likely that the sand tray itself is smaller in size and the collection of figures is limited when compared with the resources available in the office. Although humanistic sandtray therapists who provide services in-home do what is necessary to accommodate these contextual issues, we have found limitations on what can be processed in a small, portable tray compared with a standard-sized tray. Clients who have used both a portable and standard-sized tray have shared with us that they have a greater ability to include relevant themes and can more accurately depict emotional space by placing themselves further away from other family figures, for example. One solution to this issue is to encourage clients to make use of the lid of the portable tray when the space inside the tray is insufficient.

Case Study 8.15: Greg Revisited

Greg is a 44-year-old male living with his sister. Our sessions took place at Greg's day habilitation programs. During a session, Greg was asked to create a scene of his own choosing in the portable sand tray. While picking his figures, Greg quickly ran out of space in the tray. I (Robin) suggested that Greg use the sand tray lid and table as additional space, and he did. This extra space allowed for additional themes to develop that would not have happened otherwise. By making use of the portable sand tray, the sand tray lid, and the table, Greg was able to create several symbolic groupings of similar animals outside of the tray and themes of people operating businesses inside of the tray. With the use of all this space, Greg was able to accurately create a scene to communicate his theme that figures and characters have different roles and responsibilities. The creation and, therefore, processing of this theme might have been missed had Greg been forced to work within the confines of the sandtray itself. More importantly, the expanded space allowed Greg to process the pride he took in his ability to sort figures into associated groups and the success he felt at creating a cohesive world in the sandtray.

Confidentiality and Depth of Processing

Providing HST in-home, both at individual residences and group homes, or in community settings, like day habilitation programs, can increase ethical concerns about client confidentiality. Confidentiality issues arise when other individuals onsite at the therapeutic location walk through the room in which therapy is taking place or when caregivers seek out clients mid-session to provide medication or remind them of upcoming appointments. The issues with confidentiality can be mitigated by obtaining all the necessary release of information (ROI) documentation and by providing psychoeducation about the importance of confidentiality in counseling to caregivers and other individuals present onsite. However, risks to confidentiality can still impact how clients move through the HST process.

Due to the tendency of HST to bring up emotionally charged issues and the ability of HST to take clients into deep processing, it is important to take precautions to ensure confidentiality for these sessions, regardless of location. There are, however, some layers of confidentiality intrinsically present in HST, specifically because metaphor work highlights that the meaning behind the miniatures in the sandtray is initially only known to the client. In our experience, emphasizing this fact to clients provides some comfort.

Clients who benefit from HST sometimes want to share their experiences with others, which can motivate clients to invite other family members or group home members to participate in their sessions. The decision to include others in the session should be assessed on a case-by-case basis, with the determining factor being whether opening the session to additional participants would benefit the client. For example, my (Robin's) client, John (see Case Study 8.10), wanted to include his younger brother in session to show how he had benefited from HST. Specifically, John wanted to share how the sandtray could be used to tell stories. John's younger brother disregarded the instructions and stories that John was trying to share and began using the sandtray in the ways he wanted. John became frustrated and politely asked his brother to stop. John did not invite his brother to participate in future sessions. Reflecting on this session, my mistake was failing to first ask whether it would be beneficial to John if his younger brother joined the session. At this point in our therapeutic relationship, John was struggling with having his own room at his mom's house while having to share a room with his younger brother at his dad's house. There was promise in the idea that John being able to share space in the sandtray would relate to the concept of sharing space in his room at his dad's house. Despite the potential behind this idea, the exercise failed for two main reasons. I failed to realize that John's level of frustration from sharing his room had exceeded the threshold that would make sandtray sharing effective. In addition, a portable tray is too small to effectively promote sharing, regardless of the relationship dynamic of the participants.

There are also limitations placed on processing because some clients want to ensure that their session is not overheard. In our experiences, there can also be limitations placed on processing due to a client simply not wanting to bring up an issue in their home and the space in which they live. The psychological space is different when conducting sessions outside of an office. Clients no longer have the therapist's office as a place they know they can go to, discuss what is going on, and then leave. The differences in the psychological space of in-office versus in-home sessions can affect the depth and speed of process, with in-home sessions having less depth and a slower processing pace. They may have a desire to process issues while simultaneously feeling too vulnerable or exposed to do so.

Processing traumatic events outside of the office can pose a special challenge to a client due to their embarrassment or respect for their own privacy. On several occasions, we have been in the middle of processing sandtray scenes with a client when they will stop, look around, and lower their voice before continuing to talk. This series of events removes the client from the therapeutic experience and their processing. In one example, I (Robin) witnessed a client stop discussing and processing an issue of eating food that was not hers. The client knew the group home manager had cameras and did not want to accidentally incriminate herself by talking about the issue with me in session. Despite this, in-home HST can still be productive. In the in-home setting, it is important to empathize with the client's feelings about privacy.

Client Relationships with Group Home Staff

The issue of a client's relationship with their group home manager or staff comes up often when using HST in these settings. Dynamics of the relationships between clients and their group home managers vary from client to client. For some clients, the relationship with the group home manager requires tact on the part of the therapist to mitigate any potential risks for the client. For other clients, the relationship is akin to that of a parent and a child. In these cases, it is important to keep in mind that clients with disabilities who are adjusting to life with a caring group home manager often go through developmental processes related to gaining autonomy paired with seeking appropriate boundaries. Therapists working in this setting may need to make a distinction with group home managers that individuals with disabilities are not children, and a balance between autonomy and respect for boundaries needs to be negotiated. Otherwise, challenges may ensue in what can be an incredibly rewarding relationship.

Case Study 8.16: Hank

Hank is a 44-year-old male living in a group home. He has lived in several different group homes and frequently moves from one to another. Hank often talks about missing his previous group homes and group home managers. They would allow him to roam the streets at two o'clock in the morning, permit group home members to have guns in the house, and leave the group home unsupervised for extended periods of time. Hank would complain about his perceived restrictions at his new group home. He lamented the fact that he was not allowed to drive other people's cars and was frustrated by the emphasis the group home manager would place on ensuring Hank followed medical recommendations from his doctor. During HST, it became apparent that Hank's current group home manager cared deeply about him and that receiving care from a group home manager was a new experience for Hank.

In our experiences, HST can be a valuable approach to explore the relationship between the client and their group home manager. This exploration can help determine where the client is experiencing discomfort in being cared for and where the client has been hurt by mistreatment from parents and other adults who were supposed to provide guidance, respect, and love.

Humanistic Sandtray Therapy Over Time

HST can be a frontline approach to working with clients diagnosed with one or more disabilities and who struggle with overlapping complex mental health issues. Case Study 8.17 is a case example of a 13-year-old male client diagnosed with mild IDD, enuresis, depression, psychosis with an unspecified cause, auditory and visual hallucinations, ASD, Tourette's syndrome, OCD, and ADHD.

Case Study 8.17: Jason

Jason presented for trauma therapy services at the community mental health agency due to increases in aggression and self-harm when dysregulated, the frequency of spitting on and biting his mother and siblings, and difficulty processing and understanding the symptoms of his diagnoses. The escalation of Jason's challenging behaviors occurred after an alleged sexual molestation by a female relative and the onset of puberty.

During the initial assessment phase of treatment, Jason confirmed that he felt a strong desire to act aggressively toward his mother and siblings when dysregulated. He shared, however, that he experienced an intense sense of shame and guilt after acting on these aggressive tendencies. Jason described his visual hallucinations as a "dark stick figure" resembling the mind flair from the TV show *Stranger Things*. He described his auditory hallucinations as voices telling him to spit on people, to bite people, and to tell other people to "fuck off." Jason disclosed the difficulties he was facing at school. He would frequently interrupt other students, shout profanities, and display an inability to follow structured activities. He expressed feelings of shame and guilt from frequently urinating in his pants at home and at school. Jason vocalized his desire to return to the way life was before he started having difficulties.

Jason's mother shared the noticeable increases in Jason's difficult behavior since the alleged sexual molestation, and Jason's father shared the noticeable increases in Jason's difficult behavior since starting puberty. At the time, Jason's parents were in a high-conflict custody case for Jason and disagreed on a long-term solution for Jason's housing. Jason's mother wanted him to transition to a group home setting, but Jason's father wanted Jason to live at his house. Despite the disagreements and the custody case, Jason's parents worked together to ensure their son received the appropriate treatment and care. When I (Robin) began working with Jason, his parents had decided that it was no longer safe for Jason to live with his mother, and Jason had just started living with his father.

Initial Impressions

With all the resolve of a fresh-faced graduate with a brand new degree in counseling, I embarked on my therapeutic relationship with Jason holding on to the belief that what he needed was the opportunity to be a kid and to take a break from the daily life stressors brought on by school and his parents' custody case. If those things could happen, I thought Jason could then begin to process the trauma from his past and the difficulties he was currently facing at his own pace. Jason appeared to be a good candidate for play therapy, but he expressed no interest in participating in this modality. I went into our first session with the therapeutic hunch that Jason was emotionally obstructed and needed an outlet in which he could express himself and be understood.

First Session

Jason started our first session by giving a tour of his room and introducing his pet lizard. This introduction took a great deal of time as Jason slowly coaxed the lizard out from under a rock, carefully picked the lizard up, and continually told me how he wanted to make sure he did not scare or hurt his lizard friend. After introducing the lizard, Jason shared how he missed his previous therapist and was sad that he did not have a chance to say goodbye. I quickly became solution focused and encouraged Jason to write a goodbye letter to his therapist, draw his feelings, or engage in a psychodrama activity of saying goodbye. Looking back now, I recognize that I was asking too much, too soon. Jason politely declined to engage in the suggested therapeutic activities and shared that he did not think he could handle directly engaging with his sadness without being overcome by his feelings.

I had brought my portable HST kit, and the sight of a large, mysterious bag piqued Jason's interest. I opened the sandtray kit, and Jason immediately jumped into action. He felt the sand fall between his fingers, inspected the figures, and began to create his own story line. I tried to slow the process by giving Jason a prompt and providing instructions to first create a scene and then to describe the completed scene to me. Jason was too excited to hear and heed any of my instructions and requests and, instead, used the figures and sandtray to act out his own story. In that moment, I remembered and implemented my sandtray therapy training and resolved to meet Jason where he was by reflecting the emotions and themes present in his scene. The scene Jason created in our first session included themes of good, evil, danger, death, and grief and was the beginning of an epic adventure that would unfold over the course of treatment.

In our early sessions, I cautiously experimented with EMDR concepts and traditional HST approaches, including directive prompts and the defined two-step process of scene creation followed by scene processing. These experiments were met with varying success. The container exercise, an EMDR resource development concept, was effective in session two when Jason brought in a pink octopus as the dark stick figure of his visual hallucinations. At the end of the session, Jason locked the pink octopus and, by proxy, the dark stick figure in the mobile sandtray box. Jason continued to hold fast to simultaneously creating and processing a sandtray and did not implement the traditional two-step approach to HST. Also common in our early sessions was Jason's use of maladaptive self-soothing behaviors, like hitting himself on the head, banging his head, and verbally berating himself for having a verbal outburst.

In our fourth session, Jason highlighted one of the benefits of HST by using the sandtray to demonstrate what it felt like to deal with his issues and the extent of their impact on his life. Jason began this session by continuing the story he had started in the previous session and was adding figure after figure to the sandtray. He eventually dumped all of the figures into the sandtray and stated, "That's a lot of fucking shit." Through this, Jason expressed how there were a lot of things in his life that he would like to sort out, but he felt overwhelmed by the task and did not know where to start. Successfully using the sandtray to express himself in our early sessions helped Jason realize that the benefit of the sandtray was not in the figures themselves but rather in him acting out and expressing what was going on in his life with the figures. This ultimately helped him come to terms with family conflict and develop a mature understanding of good and evil.

In session ten, Jason and I found a new use for HST. The returning of responsibility was becoming a stronger theme as Jason was now able to use the sandtray to work on his own problems. After session, Jason confided in me his desire to live with his mother and to visit her more often and that he wanted to share these thoughts with his father. Jason asked me to tell his father for him. Instead, I returned the responsibility and assured Jason that he was capable of sharing this information with his father on his own. I also told Jason that he was brave and referenced the bravery demonstrated by the sandtray figures Jason chose to represent himself in his sandtray scenes. We walked from Jason's room, and Jason nervously told his father that he would like to spend more time with his mother. Jason's father was open to the concept, and they made plans to visit her that same day. While it is possible that my presence during this conversation motivated Jason's father to agree to his son's wishes, I believe it was beneficial for Jason to voluntarily face something he had been avoiding.

By session 14, Jason's emotions were being felt and experienced more freely, and Jason had started to engage in other forms of creative and expressive art. The imagination Jason employed when creating a sandtray was beginning to manifest itself in other aspects of life. He was able to differentiate between his imagination and his psychotic symptoms and could now use more traditional approaches to cope with his psychotic symptoms. What I found most impressive was the method Jason developed to differentiate between his OCD and Tourette's symptoms. Jason created a poster in which he used purple and pink pencils to create overlapping scribbles. He drew a pink line to the word "Tourette's" and a purple line to the word "OCD." Jason shared that by imagining Tourette's and OCD as colors, he could begin to untangle the thoughts and symptoms of these two distinct diagnoses and understand what was causing certain behaviors. By identifying OCD thoughts and symptoms as purple, Jason was able to focus on controlling his OCD.

In session 25, Jason dumped all of the figures into the sandtray again. This time, however, he did not express feeling overwhelmed. Instead, he smiled and sheepishly pecked at the figures in the tray. He continually returned to a police officer and a female figure and had them interact with one another by going on dates, hugging, and kissing. This led to a productive conversation in which Jason shared that there was an attractive girl in his class, and he tentatively explored the idea of pursuing a relationship with her.

In sessions 28 and 29, Jason's creativity and imagination left the confines of the sandtray as he began to incorporate stuffed animals from his room into the epic adventures of his life. For the first time, Jason was now ending our sessions with good triumphing over evil.

By session 34, Jason was exhibiting the classic signs of an adolescent ready to move on from therapy. Our sessions continually became less important to Jason while activities with his father, games with his brother, and opportunities to explore the family's new house became more important. Session 34 was our termination session, and I thought it appropriate to encourage Jason to create one last sandtray with a prompt of his choosing. With no prompting from the therapist, Jason began the scene with two knights and named them, one after himself and one after me. Jason shared that these knights would be going on one last adventure together to slay a dragon before parting ways. Jason had the two figures discuss how much they each helped the other and how, while their paths may cross again in the future, this was to be their last adventure. Jason then had the knights fight a fire-breathing dragon. The knight named after me was injured in this fight and the knight named after Jason was required to defeat the dragon on his own. Naturally, Jason beat the dragon on his own with a voice full of confidence.

Reflection

As I reflect on my work with Jason, I realize how the use of HST in our early sessions provided exactly what Jason needed. Ultimately, Jason knew what he needed more than I could have ever guessed and more than I initially gave him credit for. In my opinion, Jason illustrated how HST can help an individual with disabilities and co-occurring mental health diagnoses to develop their own freedom of expression, improve their self-esteem, self-regulate their emotions, and strengthen connections with family, friends, and caregivers.

Conclusion

Integrating HST into our clinical work with clients diagnosed with disabilities is incredibly meaningful for each of us. We have seen the powerful impacts of sandtray through both creation of client scenes and processing their new perspectives and emerging awareness. Therapists who work with this population can find great value in using HST to process everyday struggles, developmental stuck points, trauma, and relationships. Because of the wide range of client presentations and physical settings in which humanistic sandtray therapists work with their clients, we strongly recommend attending to individual adaptations of HST that allow for rich therapeutic growth.

References

American Psychiatric Association. (2022). *Diagnostic and Statistical Manual of Mental Disorders, Fifth Edition, Text Revision* (DSM-5-TR). Author.

Buhler, C. (1951). The World Test, a projective technique. *Journal of Child Psychiatry, 2*, 4–23.

Centers for Disease Control and Prevention. (2020). Disability and health promotion. https://www.cdc.gov/ncbddd/disabilityandhealth/disability-inclusion.html

Center for Substance Abuse Treatment. (2014). Trauma-informed care in behavioral health services. *Treatment Improvement Protocol (TIP) Series, No. 57.* Substance Abuse and Mental Health Services Administration. https://www.ncbi.nlm.nih.gov/books/NBK207201/

Daveny, J., Hassiotis, A., Katona, C., Matcham, F., & Sen, P. (2019). Ascertainment and prevalence of post-traumatic stress disorder (PTSD) in people with intellectual disabilities. *Journal of Mental Health Research in Intellectual Disabilities, 12*(3–4), 211–233. https://doi.org/10.1080/19315864.2019.1637979

Fried, K. (2024). Online sandtray. https://www.onlinesandtray.com

Green, J. (2013). *The fault in our stars.* Penguin Books.

Harvey, K. (2012). *Trauma-informed behavioral interventions: What works and what doesn't.* American Association on Intellectual and Developmental Disabilities.

Herman, J. L. (2022). *Trauma and recovery: The aftermath of violence—from domestic abuse to political terror.* Basic Books.

Homeyer, L. E., & Sweeney, D. S. (2023). *Sandtray therapy: A practical manual* (4th ed.). Routledge. https://doi.org/10.4324/9781003221418

Hulbert-Williams, L., Hastings, R., Owen, D. M., Burns, L., Day, J., Mulligan, J., & Noone, S. J. (2013). Exposure to life events as a risk factor for psychological problems in adults with intellectual disabilities: A longitudinal design. *Journal of Intellectual Disability Research, 58,* 48–60. http://dx.doi.org/10.1111/jir.12050

Kaufman, S. B. (2013). *Ungifted: Intelligence redefined.* Basic Books/Hachette Book Group.

Komarek, V. (2020). *"My life's been good. It changed, it's been good." The use of sandtray therapy with adults with intellectual disabilities and comorbid mental illness.* [Doctoral dissertation, Roberts Wesleyan College]. ProQuest Dissertations & Theses Global.

Larson, S., Eschenbacher, H., Anderson, L., Pettingell, S., Hewitt, A., Sowers, M., Bourne, M. L., Taylor, B., & Agosta, J. (2017). *In-home and residential long-term supports and services for persons with intellectual or developmental disabilities: Status and trends.* Institute on Community Integration. University of Minnesota. https://files.eric.ed.gov/fulltext/ED598171.pdf

Lewis, C. S. (2001). *The problem of pain.* Harper.

Marcia, J. E. (1993). *Ego identity: A handbook for psychosocial research.* Springer-Verlag.

Mevissen, L., Didden, R., de Jongh, A., & Korzilius, H. (2020). Assessing posttraumatic stress disorder in adults with mild intellectual disabilities or borderline intellectual functioning. *Journal of Mental Health Research in Intellectual Disabilities, 13*(2), 110–126. https://doi.org/10.1080/19315864.2020.1753267

Nieuwenhuis, J. G., Smits, H. J. H., Noorthoorn, E. O., Mulder, C. L., Penterman, E. J. M., & Nijman, H. L. I. (2019). Not recognized enough: The effects and associations of trauma and intellectual disability in severely mentally ill outpatients. *European Psychiatry, 58,* 63–69. https://doi.org/10.1016/j.eurpsy.2019.02.002

Presnell, J., Keesler, J. M., & Thomas-Giyer, J. (2022). Assessing alignment between intellectual and developmental disability service providers and trauma-informed care: An exploratory study. *Intellectual and Developmental Disabilities, 60*(5), 351–368. https://doi.org/10.1352/1934-9556-60.5.351

Scotti, J. R., Stevens, S. B., Jacoby, V. M., Bracken, M. R., Freed, R., & Schmidt, E. (2012). Trauma in people with intellectual and developmental disabilities: Reactions of parents and caregivers to research participation. *Intellectual and Developmental Disabilities, 50*(3), 199–206. http://dx.doi.org/10.1352/1934-9556-50.3.199

Sevcik, R. A., Barton-Hulsey, A., Bruce, S., Goldman, A., Ogletree, B. T., Paul, D., & Romski, M. (2022). It's never too late: Debunking myths about communication and adults with severe disabilities. *Intellectual and Developmental Disabilities, 60*(5), 416-425. https://doi.org/10.1352/1934-9556-60.5.416

Shapiro, F. (2017). *Eye movement desensitization and reprocessing (EMDR) therapy: Basic principles, protocols and procedures* (3rd ed.). Guilford Press.

Shew, A. (2023). *Against technoableism: Rethinking who needs improvement.* W. W. Norton & Company.

Smith, S. D. (2012). *Sandtray play and storymaking: A hands-on approach to build academic, social, and emotional skills in mainstream and special education.* Jessica Kingsley.

Tanguay, D. (2009). Adapting sandtray assessment for adults with developmental disabilities. In S. Snow & M. D'Amico (Eds.), *Assessment in the creative arts therapies: Designing and adapting assessment tools for adults with developmental disabilities* (pp. 219–256). Charles C. Thomas.

U.S. Department of Justice Civil Rights Division. (2010). ADA standards for accessible design. https://www.ada.gov/law-and-regs/design-standards/

Part III

Clinical Applications and Settings

Chapter 9

Humanistic Sandtray Therapy in Group Work

Counseling and psychotherapy groups are an excellent clinical situation for HST. Homeyer and Sweeney (2023) outlined advantageous characteristics of sandtray groups, including group member spontaneity, an emphasis on emotional experiencing, exposure to vicarious learning via observations of other group members' patterns of emotional responses, a focus on self-exploration, concentration on the here and now, and development of inter-personal relationship skills. Although many of these qualities overlap with group work generally, sandtray can be a powerful way of encouraging con-tact and inclusion among group members. Sandtray groups can assist group members to increase their awareness of boundaries and contact boundary disturbances in ways that individual therapy cannot, due to opportunities for interpersonal conflict development, resolution, peer validation, and group modeling, all elements inherent to group dynamics.

Clinicians can integrate HST into group work in two primary ways: using sandtray as an experiment from time to time in a group or running a sandtray group in which group members create sandtrays during every ses-sion. You can use the information in this chapter in either scenario. Of course, when creating a group, it is important to ensure that sandtray fits within the group's goals as well as the overall personality of the group. HST can act to get group members involved in ways that are not likely in a typical talk therapy group. It can also be a good adjunct to existing groups in which sandtray is not the primary vehicle of processing. In this chapter, my goals are to provide you with practical guidance regarding use of sandtray in groups and to review how HST fits into established principles of group work.

Developmental Considerations

HST can be used with groups that include members across the age spec-trum from preadolescents to adults. Bratton and Ferebee (1999) stated that sandtray gives preadolescent group members "opportunities to change

DOI: 10.4324/9781032664996-12

perceptions about self, others and the world" (p. 193). Armstrong, Foster, and Hickman (2022) described HST in preadolescent groups. They acknowledged that preadolescent and young adolescent HST groups can be a powerful growth experience due to wide applicability during a developmental period that is in between concrete and abstract thinking. Because group members may vary significantly in terms of development even when they are the same age, HST can be a unifying experience. Expressive arts attune to preadolescents' and young adolescents' natural modes of communication, combining verbal and non-verbal methods.

For older adolescent and adult groups, HST can tune in to members' abstract thinking abilities wherein the trays can provide a safe medium for group members to get to know each other, process their intragroup and intrapersonal conflicts, and become productive groups. It is important for humanistic sandtray therapists to attune to safety and trust in groups when using sandtray in earlier group phases, which I will discuss later in this chapter. However, I encourage humanistic sandtray group leaders to provide cautious sandtray prompts when members are getting to know each other. In addition, I recommend leaning into a person-centered facilitative mode in earlier phases of older adolescent and adult groups until a degree of intragroup trust is established.

Practical Considerations

Because there are so many possibilities for HST in group work, I recommend that you put some thought into what is practical for you and your groups. If you are anything like me, you might dream big but then get hit with the reality of your miniatures collection, your clinical space, and your access to multiple sand trays. Think about what is reasonable given your clinical context, client needs, and the sandtray materials that are available to you. Some clinical context considerations include:

- Are you using sandtray as one among many expressive arts media in your group? Or are you going to facilitate a sandtray group, in which sandtray is the primary mode of expression?
- How many group members do you plan to have? Although six to eight group members is the "magic number" to create an effective group for adolescents and adults (Corey, 2022), Flahive and Ray (2007) recommended that preadolescent sandtray groups consist of a maximum of four members. Will you be able to accommodate this many group members given your clinical space and time allotment?
- Will you prompt group members to create individual trays? Group trays? Both?

Depending on your answers to the questions above, you will need to ensure that you have enough sandtray materials, an adequate physical space, and a sufficient time allotment for the group to work well. When thinking about miniatures, I highly recommend that you have multiple copies of almost all of them. Although this may not be possible for some of the unique miniatures in your collection, it is wise for you to make this suggestion a guiding standard. Clients should have relatively equal access to miniatures. Of course, complying with this guideline will require significant financial investment on your part.

In addition to miniatures, the kinds of sand trays you have will be impacted by your approach to the group; that is, whether group members will construct individual trays, a group tray, or a mix. For individual trays, you may want to consider smaller, portable trays. However, a limitation to smaller trays is that it limits the client's expressivity—a few of my clients with whom I have used portable trays have voiced this issue to me. If you plan to facilitate a group tray, wherein all your group members work in one sand tray, Homeyer and Sweeney (2023) have step-by-step instructions that you could use to build your own larger tray with sufficient dimensions. Another way I have facilitated groups is with larger adult groups of around 12 members. I randomly put them into smaller groups of four members, each using one standard-sized tray, and prompted them to create a scene in the tray so that there were three trays to share in the group.

A final practical consideration is the physical setting in which you host your group. I recommend that you have enough room for members to move around and select figures, just as you would in individual HST. As you might imagine, you will need a pretty large room to accommodate this guideline. Finally, when doing sandtray in groups, I have found that using tables instead of shelves to display miniatures allows group members to access the miniatures more freely. An easy way to categorize miniatures when using tables is to arrange them into clear plastic bins, which can be bought at dollar stores. Ensure that the bins are not overflowing and that all of the figures are visible. I have made the mistake of overfilling those containers and watching group members rifle through them to find the miniatures they want.

Principles of Group Work

Group work is a field that requires specialization and focused training (Association for Specialists in Group Work, 2021). The group experience pushes and pulls group members and leaders in ways that they may not have been exposed to before. A prerequisite for integrating HST into group work is that the practitioner has notable experience leading groups and has depth of knowledge and understanding of the major principles that underlie group work. Although it is beyond the scope of this book to discuss every element of putting together a group, standardizing the group, and best practices, there are a few principles of group work that I will discuss from an HST point of view: Yalom and Leszcz's (2005) therapeutic factors, group phases (Tuckman, 1965; Tuckman & Jensen, 1977), and Luft's (1969) Johari window.

Therapeutic Factors

Yalom and Leszcz (2005) noted 11 therapeutic factors of group work that have meaningful application to HST. According to Yalom and Leszcz, these therapeutic factors—also known as curative factors—represent the heart of change in a group: "an enormously complex process that occurs through an interplay of human experiences" (p. 1). These factors cannot be separated and intertwine as group members interact as a whole and as individual members. From my point of view, HST can act as a mediator of these processes when applied to group work. In other words, group members' sandtray scenes as well as the processing phase of group HST can facilitate these factors.

Yalom and Leszcz (2005) noted four factors that were most influenced by the group leader, known as therapist factors:

- *Instillation of hope*: Group leaders have a responsibility to provide optimism. When humanistic sandtray therapists adopt an attitude in groups based on the belief that people have innate mechanisms that move them toward growth and actualization, it can be therapeutic to members because they have the opportunity to introject a hopeful outlook.
- *Universality*: Pain, hurt, and suffering can entice individual group members to believe that they are alone in their experiences. On the contrary, sandtray scenes can provide a stark visual image to group members that they are not unique in their misery.
- *Imparting of information*: Yalom and Leszcz (2005) suggested that didactic education can be useful in groups, particularly when group goals are concrete in nature. Although this concept could be misinterpreted by the humanistic sandtray therapist as providing "shoulds" to group members, members are exposed to direct learning by observation of skills intended to increase awareness. For example, inviting group members to do bodywork is a way of imparting information in which the goal is to assist clients in practices designed for self-awareness.
- *Altruism*: Group leaders have a responsibility to model valuing of each group member and what members can give each other. Leaders demonstrate that reciprocal giving and receiving is not the only way to heal; acts of giving to others without an expectation of reciprocity can be

therapeutic. In HST groups, humanistic group leaders model empathy, presence, and compassion and exemplify transcendence of self in service of others in ways that group members then begin doing for each other.

The remaining seven factors are client factors (Yalom & Leszcz, 2005), which are most influenced by group members as well as the group as a collective:

- *Corrective recapitulation of the primary family group*: Groups exhibit similar dynamics as family systems with associated subsystems. There are parental figures, siblings, and polarized emotional experiencing. Group members tend to assume roles and dynamics reflective of their families of origin. HST groups can lean into this therapeutic factor by exploring members' here-and-now experiencing of self and others, leading to the discovery of individual member polarities. In addition, as unfinished business arises in members' foreground of experiencing, HST processing provides space to begin completing members' gestalts by first completing gestalts that happen in the immediacy of the group.
- *Development of socializing techniques*: All groups provide members with direct and indirect ways of observing interpersonal processes and skills. Because HST is seated in the here and now, members demonstrate to each other habits of socializing that either lead to conflicts, and thus conflict resolution, or increased closeness.
- *Imitative behavior*: Because group members observe and influence each other directly and indirectly, they begin to experiment with enacting what they have learned. In HST, a group member's behavior may symbolize another member's disowned part and provide an opportunity to enact that part.
- *Interpersonal learning*: Groups highlight the gestalt principle that people do not operate outside of their environment or situation and healthy interpersonal relationships are necessary for growth. Yalom and Leszcz (2005) described the important role of corrective emotional experiences in group work. In HST, a partner process to increased awareness is risk taking, and supportive groups provide members with an impetus to try to succeed, or fail and try something different.
- *Group cohesiveness*: This factor is a precondition for all other therapeutic factors. Cohesiveness provides members with a safe home that mirrors unconditional positive regard, warmth, and valuing. When HST groups arrive at a sense of cohesiveness, members feel safe enough to consider change.
- *Catharsis*: Although catharsis is not enough on its own for group members to change, it can be a therapeutic experience that leads to contact, inclusion, and cohesiveness in HST groups.

- *Existential factors*: As a person-centered gestaltist approach, HST is strongly influenced by existentialism. It is common for HST group members to symbolize existential themes in their trays, and groups highlight the universality of these factors as members see each other struggle with the same underlying truths of existence: life is not always fair or just; pain and death are inevitable; people live life internally alone regardless of the degree of intimacy they have with others; ultimately, people's search for meaning is best accomplished with authenticity; and because people face consequences of their life decisions alone, they are responsible fundamentally for their own conduct.

Group Phases

Groups tend to progress following a trajectory outlined by Tuckman (1965) and Tuckman and Jensen (1977) based on their systematic reviews of small group functioning. Famously known as forming, storming, norming, performing, and adjourning, they are better described as phases because groups may stagnate in one place and never progress or regress temporarily (or permanently). Each group is a unique collective, and I would recommend viewing these developmental phases as guidelines rather than rigid categories. If you treat these as expectations for your groups, then all you are doing is projecting shouldistic regulation. Despite these caveats, conceptualizing progression of HST groups as one might view formation and maintenance of any organization or system helps humanistic sandtray therapists to know practical elements such as what kind of group prompts might be appropriate in response to the phase in which the group appears to be operating.

During the *forming* phase, members are getting to know each other and the group leader (Tuckman, 1965; Tuckman & Jensen, 1977). The group leader typically works with members to establish group rules and procedures. Members tend to experience anxiety and usually process surface issues. You may want to use HST as an experiment designed to help group members get to know each other and touch on individual and group goals. Here are a few prompts that you can use whether you are leading an HST group or using sandtray as an experiment during a group session in the forming phase:

- "Create a world that helps others know who you are. You could include likes, dislikes, wishes, hopes, and challenges" (Armstrong et al., 2022, p. 33).
- Create a scene that communicates what you would like to get out of the group.
- Create a scene that lets others in the group know what is most important to know about you.

The next phase, storming, is characterized by conflict and turbulence (Tuckman, 1965; Tuckman & Jensen, 1977). The group is working through establishing their inner "hierarchy" by partnering with anxiety and power struggles. Sometimes, one or more members attack the group leader as a symbol of ultimate authority. How the group navigates the storming phase often becomes the blueprint for the rest of the group experience. HST can be used to help the group confront their intragroup disorder and co-create conflict resolutions. Following are some sandtray prompts that align with the storming phase:

- "Build a scene in the sand that shows how you see yourself and your group members" (Armstrong et al., 2022, p. 33).
- Using either one large sand tray that group members all use together, or randomly splitting group members into teams to use a standard-sized tray, instruct them to create a tray without talking. You can use any number of prompts here. The point here is to observe their non-verbal communication strategies and conflict management styles.
- Create a scene that depicts the biggest hurdles to your trust in the group.
- Create a world in which the group has resolved its major conflicts.

The third phase of group development is *norming* (Tuckman, 1965; Tuckman & Jensen, 1977). When the group survives the storming phase, they experience a sense of cohesiveness and optimism. Although groups are still relationally fragile during this phase, they have become more goal-oriented and focused on problem-solving (Saidla, 1990). A qualitative difference between the norming phase and earlier phases is evident in the significant trust that members place in the process, each other, and the group leader. Here are a few prompts you may consider using during the norming phase:

- "Using any of the miniatures you'd like, make a scene that depicts your favorite problem-solving tools" (Armstrong et al., 2022, p. 34).
- Create a scene about how you see trust in this group.
- Create a scene about this group's identity and how you fit with it.

Next is the performing phase, known as the working phase (Tuckman, 1965; Tuckman & Jensen, 1977). Trust and cohesiveness are at an all-time high. Group members take risks more frequently because they feel supported and accepted by each other. HST can have an important place during the performing phase as it can be used as experimentation to facilitate risk-taking, conflict resolution, or to validate members' experiences. Some example prompts that can be used during this phase are:

- "[C]reate a scene in the sandtray about how [you] see each others' worlds" (Armstrong et al., 2022, p. 34).
- Build a scene in the sand that expresses a need that you're experiencing right now.
- Create a world in which you feel free to expose your greatest fears.
- Create a scene about your group connection.

Tuckman and Jensen's (1977) fifth stage of *adjourning* is tantamount to group termination. Group members say goodbye to each other, the group as a collective, and the process. HST can assist in the termination process to help members reflect on how much they have grown, their wishes for the future, and to provide a good gestalt for the group experience. Here are a few prompts I suggest during this phase:

- "Make a scene in the sandtray that shows how you have seen yourself change" (Armstrong et al., 2022, p. 34).
- "Make a scene that shows others how you feel about ending the group" (Armstrong et al., 2022, p. 34).
- Create a scene that communicates your experience of this group.
- Create a world that captures how you have made meaning of your group experience.

Interpersonal Behavior and Awareness in Groups

A final group principle worth noting is based on the Johari window (Luft, 1969), which is a way of understanding interpersonal behavior and awareness. Shakoor (2010) described his application of the Johari window to group work. The Johari window arranges people's awareness of their emotions, behaviors, and motivations on a continuum of aware–unaware by placing this process on a 2 × 2 four-quadrant model. Luft (1969) labeled the top quadrants as Q-1 Open and Q-2 Blind, and the bottom quadrants as Q-3 Hidden and Q-4 Unknown.

Q-1 captures emotions, behaviors, and motivations that are known to self and to others (Luft, 1969). Shakoor (2010) stated that one goal of group work is for group members to grow this quadrant. In other words, group can act as a way for members to increase awareness of self and to communicate this awareness to others. This goal aligns seamlessly with HST. Some scenes, especially early sandtrays in a group, fit into this quadrant on a surface level. As the group moves into the storming phase, the ability of group members to begin to open up the flow of this quadrant and enlarge it will be the task at hand.

Q-2 represents emotions, behaviors, and motivations that are unknown to self and known to others (Luft, 1969). Shakoor (2010) believed that assuming a discovery-oriented and risk-taking position was a central Q-2 challenge for group members. HST can be a guidepost for group members in this regard, and one way group leaders can facilitate shrinking group members' blind areas is to provide sandtray prompts that illuminate how group members perceive each other.

Q-3 denotes emotions, behaviors, and motivations that are known to self and unknown to others (Luft, 1969). These are aspects of self that people keep hidden intentionally from others. Shakoor (2010) noted that "[d]isclosures from Q-3 help you to be seen more clearly and leave you with less to hide" (p. xviii) and immediately transmit these hidden aspects to Q-1. A meaningful function of HST in group work is to facilitate the disclosure of Q-3 self-data to Q-1, thereby allowing other group members to experience and know each other. Using individual trays along with prompts designed to elicit member self-disclosure during group work is one way to invite them into this experience.

Finally, Q-4 represents emotions, behaviors, and motivations that are unknown to self and others (Luft, 1969). As groups move through later phases, particularly norming and performing, members will discover self-data that was previously unknown and shifts into another quadrant (Shakoor, 2010). Sometimes this unknown-to-all data becomes known to self first and sometimes to others first. In either case, it can be a jolting experience for group members. Because HST is an exploration and discovery-oriented process, it may act as a window to shift Q-4 information and experiencing to become known. When members experience these shifts during HST group work, it is essential for the group leader to lean into a person-centered mode of warmth, unconditional positive regard, empathy, authenticity, and acceptance.

Conclusion

Applying HST to counseling and psychotherapy groups can provide a deeply transformative experience for members and leader alike. Because HST is a flexible approach designed to accommodate client needs, it can be used with preadolescent, adolescent, and adult groups. Sandtray in groups requires a notable upfront investment in materials and clinical space; however, HST is responsive across group phases, facilitating therapeutic factors and providing a safe medium for group member discovery and disclosure.

References

Armstrong, S. A., Foster, R. D., & Hickman, D. L. (2022). Humanistic sandtray with preadolescent groups. In C. Mellenthin, J. Stone, & R. J. Grant (Eds.), *Implementing play therapy with groups: Contemporary issues in practice* (pp. 26–38). Routledge.

Association for Specialists in Group Work. (2021). *Guiding principles for group work.* https://asgw.org/wp-content/uploads/2021/07/ASGW-Guiding-Principles-May-2021.pdf

Bratton, S., & Ferebee, K. (1999). The use of structured expressive art activities in group activity therapy for preadolescents. In D. S. Sweeney & L. E. Homeyer (Eds.), *The handbook of group play therapy: How to do it, how it works, whom it's best for* (pp. 192–214). Jossey-Bass.

Corey, G. (2022). *Theory and practice of group counseling* (10th ed.). Cengage.

Flahive, M. W., & Ray, D. (2007). Effect of group sandtray therapy with preadolescents. *Journal for Specialists in Group Work, 32,* 362–382. https://doi.org/10.1080/01933920701476706

Homeyer, L. E., & Sweeney, D. S. (2023). *Sandtray therapy: A practical manual* (4th ed.). Routledge.

Luft, J. (1969). *Of human interaction.* National Press.

Saidla, D. D. (1990). Cognitive development and group stages. *The Journal for Specialists in Group Work, 15*(1), 15–20. http://dx.doi.org/10.1080/01933929008411907

Shakoor, M. (2010). *On becoming a group member: Personal growth and effectiveness in group counseling.* Routledge.

Tuckman, B. W. (1965). Developmental sequence in small groups. *Psychological Bulletin, 63*(6), 384–399. https://doi.org/10.1037%2Fh0022100

Tuckman, B. W., & Jensen, M. A. (1977). Stages of small-group development revisited. *Group & Organization Studies, 2*(4), 419–427. https://doi.org/10.1177/105960117700200404

Yalom, I. D., & Leszcz, M. (2005). *The theory and practice of group psychotherapy* (5th ed.). Basic Books.

Chapter 10

Humanistic Sandtray Therapy with Couples and Families

Experiential work has a long history in couples and family therapy. Satir (1983) is famous for employing family sculpting to create awareness of positioning, dynamics, and hidden emotion in families, and Whitaker (Whitaker & Keith, 1981) suggested to families that they become as "crazy" as he acted in order to bring out their inner capacities for reorganization, growth, and healing. I have used several expressive arts media in my clinical work with couples and families, but my favorite (predictably) is sandtray. In my experience, sandtray can make complexities of intrapsychic wounds, relational dynamics, and systemic unfinished business so much clearer than talk therapy. HST really does get to the hearts of the matter. I would never say that HST is *better* than other approaches; however, it tends to simplify the work. Notice I said *simplify*—it does not make couples and family work any *easier*!

Although this chapter combines couples and family work, they are indeed different enterprises requiring specialized training and experience. Homeyer and Sweeney (2023) stressed the importance of dual training in sandtray and couples and/or family therapy. I echo their assertion and suggest that HST can be a good adjunct to couples and family therapy. In family therapy, sandtray can help to place family members of different ages and developmental levels on equitable communication footing (Sweeney & Rocha, 2000). In couples therapy, I have witnessed how HST can uniquely allow partners to see each other's perceptions and worlds in ways that can be captured beyond words. In this chapter, I aim to summarize theoretical elements of HST in couples and family therapy. I will also discuss practical, structural, and process considerations when integrating HST in systems work.

Theoretical Elements of HST with Couples and Families

To successfully integrate HST into couples and family therapy, humanistic sandtray therapists maintain their person-centered gestaltist philosophy.

DOI: 10.4324/9781032664996-13

Zinker (1994/1998) described gestalt as a systems theory, with its roots in holism. Couples and families are systems with internal boundaries—as well as boundaries between the system and its environment (e.g., the community). System boundaries operate on the same spectrum of permeability as individual boundaries. Zinker defined a well-functioning family as one that has "fluid, flexible subsystem boundaries among individuals and groupings of adults and children .... There is a common purpose, solidarity, cohesiveness, and responsiveness, as well as a respect for each person's separateness and specialness" (p. 53). Unhealthy family and couple systems have either overly permeable or impermeable boundaries between individuals in the system and with the environment. Families or couples with impermeable boundaries between the system and the environment are termed *retroflected families*, and families or couples with too permeable boundaries between the system and the environment are termed *disorganized families*. Zinker believed that no one subsystem or individual could be blamed and that finding a causal factor was a hopeless endeavor and argued for viewing systems as complex wholes. He saw working with couples and families as a holistic approach in which "the therapist's sense of metaphor and creative imagery will help make it possible to find the patterns of the larger organism" (p. 58). Although Zinker's approach to couples and family therapy is aligned with systems theories in general, the specifics of a gestalt approach strengthen the therapist's reliance on process rather than content.

One important theoretical concept of HST is the cycle of experience (see Chapter 1). Humanistic sandtray therapists view couples and families through this same lens, although shifted a bit to observe familiar relational interactions in the system. Observing these interactions requires attuning to individual cycles of experience as well as how these cycles of experience are interactional (Zinker, 1994/1998). In the first phase of the cycle, awareness, HST therapists observe how individuals in the system disclose self to other(s), how the other(s) respond(s), and the dynamic interplay of communication. HST therapists also attend to any resistances to awareness that arise. Awareness in systems is related to how others attune to each other, listen to each other, and respond with a new self-disclosure. During the action phase of the cycle, couples and families will have competing wants, interests, and needs. Systems that function well are composed of individuals who are able to manage differences so that the individuals invest in owning clearly these needs, wants, and interests as a system. Next, during contact, couples and families experience a sensation of ownership of the common wants and needs. Finally, during the satisfaction phase, the couple or family system "summarizes, reflects, and savors the experience, then nails it down" (p. 75).

Moreover, Zinker (1994/1998) outlined various roles of couples and family therapists. HST complements these roles as noted below:

- The therapist works with systems to observe their own interactional process. HST can be used here as a method for couples and families to notice how they construct their trays, whether they create individual or joint scenes. Humanistic sandtray therapists identify any resistances that they observe during the creation and processing phases of HST.
- Therapists structure sessions in ways that facilitate individuals in couples or families to "interact directly with each other, rather than focusing their attention on the clinicians" (p. 84). Therefore, humanistic sandtray therapists invite couples or family members to talk to each other during the processing phase of HST. For example, instead of asking a family member, "What is it like to create your sandtray scene?" I would say, "Mom, tell your family what it is like to create your sandtray scene." This gives me the opportunity to observe the family's cycle of experience.
- Therapists propose experiments that allow couples and families to increase their here-and-now awareness in novel situations. Zinker stated that increased awareness leads couples and families to "enlarge their competence" (p. 85), which is another way to say that awareness exposes people to choices they did not realize they had and have new avenues for behavioral change. HST can be one such experiment.
- Therapists apply polarities work, a keystone of HST processing.

Therapists who have training and clinical experience with HST as well as couples and family therapy are prepared to merge these approaches to provide clients with a creative, spontaneous, and grounded healing experience.

Practical Considerations

As you know by now, humanistic sandtray therapists prepare themselves to work with their population of choice by investing intentionally in sandtray materials. I will begin by talking about miniatures. When working with couples and families, similar to working with groups, it is a good idea to have multiple copies of most of your miniatures. You do not need to have multiple copies of all miniatures, but you want to think about having "families" of miniatures. For example, when you buy animal miniatures, make sure to have animals who can represent at least a two-caregiver household—although it is a good idea to have more than two because of the diversity of family structures (e.g., for clients whose grandparents are important caregivers as well as their primary caregivers). So, instead of one adult elephant miniature, think about having three to four, and several sizes of elephants to represent children. I encourage you to apply these guidelines to other categories of miniatures as well, such as trees or flowers. What will help you is to think systemically and consider coupled items and family items. Along the same lines, be sure to have miniatures that can represent different kinds of families and couples based on sexual or affectional orientation, relationship configurations, gender identity, racial and ethnic identity, disability, and indigenous status. Take into consideration that the term "couple" does not need to mean two people—you may have a polyamorous "couple" of three or four partners. In other words, use the ADDRESSING model (Hays, 2022) to guide your collection but think about it on a systems level rather than an individual level.

Another consideration regards time. For a couples sandtray session, I recommend that you schedule at least a 90-minute session. Usually this is adequate time for the creation and processing phases. For family sandtray sessions, I recommend anywhere from two to three hours, depending on the size of the family. I can almost hear your reaction to reading "three hours" ("In what world is this academic living?")—but it may mean you meet every other week. If it is a family of three to four people, then two hours may be sufficient. Ensuring that every member in a couple or family has a chance to describe their trays and respond to others is vital.

My practical considerations regarding sand trays and physical space are similar to my discussion in Chapter 9. I will talk more about using individual and joint sandtray prompts later in this chapter. When thinking about trays, you will want to have access to as many trays as you have individuals in session. I once saw a blended family of seven people and, unfortunately, did not have access to seven trays, so I used other expressive arts activities instead of HST. I would estimate having ten trays accessible to you is ideal. Of course, for most therapy practices, this would mean you would use portable sand trays. For couples, I recommend that you invest in two standard-sized trays. Avoid splitting a standard-sized tray in half with a divider because in HST, you want to observe how the couples non-verbally interact, including how they position their sand trays (close together or far apart?) and their body positioning toward or away from each other. I will talk more about these interpersonal dynamics in the next section.

Structure and Process Considerations

Couples and family therapy can be overwhelming for therapists and clients alike. Emotions often run high, and because humanistic sandtray therapists focus on here-and-now awareness, the tension in the room can be heavy. Therapist confidence, congruence, presence, and spontaneity are significant factors for therapeutic progress. Therefore, it is important to entertain how multidimensional complexities in systems require humanistic sandtray therapists to remain grounded in their work, lest they confluence with destabilizing system dynamics. There are three major structure and process considerations in HST with couples and families that I am going to discuss: clinical rationale for individual and joint trays; responding in a facilitative and discovery-oriented manner to the system; and system polarities and resistance.

Individual and Joint Trays

Homeyer and Sweeney (2023) stated that they typically start off using individual trays with couples and families before facilitating a joint sandtray session, and I integrate this concept into HST as well. Members of couples and families usually arrive at therapy feeling unheard and unseen within their systems, and prompting them to do individual trays as their first sandtray experience allows them to express themselves in an environment that is structured for therapists to hear and see them and coach others in the process of seeing and hearing each other. In addition, facilitating individual trays invites far more safety than joint trays in the beginning phases of therapy. There are different ways to prompt and structure individual and joint trays when working with couples versus families and I discuss these varieties next.

Couples

Zinker (1994/1998) recommended that observing couples' existing interactional process is fundamental to getting to know the system. During the creation phase, humanistic sandtray therapists take the same approach as with individuals—remain silent unless a client says something to you and make your response brief. Observe their process of creation. How close do they stand to each other as they look at the miniatures? If one of the partners is standing in front of a miniature that the other wants, how do they negotiate that? What happens when each partner wants the same miniature, and you only have one? If they are making a joint tray, how is their scene mapped out in the sand—are they making one whole scene, or two mini scenes? These observational inquiries are important to note as you build a conceptual understanding of their cycle of experience, boundaries, and contact disturbances.

In terms of sandtray prompts, Homeyer and Sweeney (2023) provide some in their appendix that can be useful for couples and families. In addition to those, here are some prompts to use when couples are creating individual trays:

- Create a scene that describes how you view your relationship.
- Create a scene about the major problems in your relationship as you see them.
- Create a scene that tells your partner who you are, including the parts you hide from them.
- Create a scene that shows how you think your partner perceives you.

Once you have had two or three sessions of individual trays, then you can move into joint sandtrays. There are a couple of strategies that you can use with joint trays. One strategy is to allow couples to talk to each other while they construct their tray; the other is to set a ground rule that they may not talk while creating their tray. Be intentional about how you set up joint trays. The second strategy is especially useful if you want to observe their non-verbal and relational dynamics while they work together on a shared task. Here are some example prompts to use for a joint sand tray:

• Create a scene that shows a typical day that you spend together.
• Make a world in which you both feel fulfilled together.
• Create a scene that expresses your shared relationship values.
• Create a scene about the moment you met each other for the first time.

During the processing phase, the therapist should have partners talk to each other. I recommend going one step further and encourage them to face each other (see Figure 10.1); this positioning helps clients avoid defaulting to talking through the therapist. While observing their process, the therapist may interrupt them to point out something they may think is valuable to the couple. I will talk more about facilitative skills during the processing phase later in this chapter.

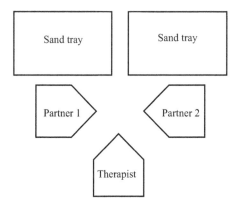

Figure 10.1 Therapist and a couple using two individual sand trays.

Families

Things typically move more quickly in family therapy, so observation of process can be more difficult (Zinker, 1994/1998). However, HST can slow things down a bit. Instead of families arguing about their differing perceptions about a situation, they can see each other's differences in individual trays. Instead of arguing about the adolescent's curfew and skipping school, they can recreate their habitual conflict patterns while constructing a joint family sandtray. HST can also help family members make their emotional experiencing clearer. The humanistic sandtray therapist's role when working with families is like working with couples in terms of observation of their relational dynamics during the creation phase; however, sandtray prompts will vary with families who include children and/or adolescents in different developmental phases. Following are prompts for creating individual trays in family HST:

- Construct "a typical day in the life of our family household" in the tray.
- Create a scene about your sense of belonging in your family.
- Create a scene of what you like about your family.
- Create a scene of what you dislike about your family.
- Create a scene about whom you feel closest to in your family.
- Create a scene about whom you feel most distant from in your family.

I advise that after one or two sessions of individual trays you can invite them to create a joint tray. Here are some example prompts for joint family sand trays:

- Without talking to each other, create a scene about your favorite thing to do together as a family.
- Create a map of your house and where people typically spend their time. Make sure everyone is doing something in the scene.

When entering the processing phase of HST, arrange family members in a way that they are facing each other. Ensure that, when they discuss their scenes, that they are talking to each other rather than to the therapist. Like couples HST, the therapist can interrupt to point out family habits of inter-action, emotional responses, and dynamics.

Facilitative Responses to the System

It is easy to forget the role of a humanistic sandtray therapist during couples and family therapy. Couples and families typically present to therapy as a last attempt at resolving their issues. Therefore, they want the therapist to be the expert, align with each of their views, rally the troops against the "problem" individual, and solve their problems for them. Of course, these aspects are not true of every couple or family. However, they are more common than not. The risk of therapist confluence with the system is elevated. Remember, even with couples and families, the humanistic sandtray therapist's role is to invite the individuals and the system into a process of discovery, explor-ation, and awareness. Use reflection of feelings liberally. Apply the HST *guiding into–staying with–going deeper into emotional experiencing* model presented in Chapter 4 as the default process with couples and families. The facilitative responses that humanistic sandtray therapists provide remain the same with an explicit focus on awareness and paradoxical change.

Case Study 10.1: Maya and Will

Maya and Will were a married heterosexual couple. They were married a little under one year when I saw them for an HST session. Will had experienced multiple sandtrays with his therapist in the past, and this was Maya's first sandtray experience. She remarked that she had heard a lot about sandtray from Will and was curious about it. They presented with wanting to explore their relationship and each other. After engaging in a centering exercise, I asked them each to create individual sandtrays, and each used a standard-sized tray. I gave them the following prompt: "Create a scene about how you view your relationship now. There may be elements of the past or the future but try to focus on your perception of your relationship now." What I am going to describe is a portion of our session together.

During the creation phase, Maya and Will seemed invested in making their autonomous sandtray scenes. I noticed each partner selected their miniatures carefully and arranged them thoughtfully in the sand. When they signaled that they were finished with their individual scenes, I asked them to turn to face each other and describe what it was like to create their scenes. Maya spoke first and stated that creating her scene connected her to herself in a way that felt unexpected. She naturally began to describe her scene (see Figure 10.2). She stated that she and Will were standing together along with Jesus Christ behind three bridges, which symbolized different paths for the future of their marriage. One path involved continuing to nurture their careers, another path involved having children and creating a family, and yet another represented nesting together as a couple and really investing in their intimate relationship. She stated that she was confused about which path Will saw as most important for them to begin to head toward in the short term. She said that sometimes her confusion led them to having arguments. I reflected her feelings of safety attached to having a plan for the future because it indicated security to her. She affirmed my reflection.

I turned to Will and asked him to describe his reaction to Maya's sandtray scene. He stated that he valued her perspective and said that he thinks their trays were connected. Then, Will described a major feature of his tray (see Figure 10.2). He had placed a figure representing himself inside of a hut. He stated that sometimes he stays hidden inside of the hut because he was afraid that if he fully exited his safe place then he might be rejected by Maya. A figure representing her was standing right outside of the hut. He also included bridge symbology.

I asked Maya to describe her reaction to Will's discussion of his tray and his perceptions of self and their relationship. She stated that she was surprised and also felt sad that he experienced such hesitation and fear about being vulnerable with her. I encouraged her to face him and tell him what she just told me. I noticed that she was tearful as she spoke, and Will also began to feel a sense of vulnerability and openness toward her. They each expressed feeling a sense of love and value from each other as they both reached out to hold each other's hands.

After further processing, I encouraged them to tell their partner what they have learned about each other during this sandtray process. They expressed that they got a deeper look into the other's wishes and fears and also felt a sense of relational intimacy with each other. They each stated how powerful the sandtray experience was for them. Maya stated that she was able to see not only her own world but also was able to view Will's world from his point of view. They both reflected that they were far more similar in how they viewed their relationship than dissimilar, and this realization felt encouraging.

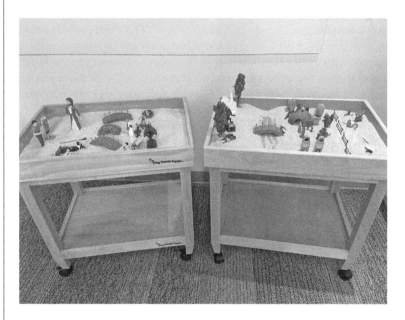

Figure 10.2 Maya's sandtray (left) and Will's sandtray (right).

Polarities and Resistance

Two major interpersonal dynamics are at play during couples and family work, just as they are in individual HST: polarities and resistance. In HST, these processes emerge within individuals in the system and as a systemic response. In other words, therapists will be able to observe multiple levels of polarities and resistance. For example, I once counseled a heterosexual married couple, Jamie and Doug, whose process of working out disagreements looked something like this: Jamie would bring an issue up to Doug. Doug carried anxiety most of the time but was usually unaware of the degree of his anxiety; therefore, Doug's anxiety about feeling confronted would rise rapidly and he would often react to Jamie with irritation. Jamie would, in turn, become angry and raise her voice. Doug would feel scared—again, out of his immediate awareness—and make efforts to shut down the conversation either by "giving in" to Jamie's request or by trying to convince Jamie to delay their discussion or decision-making process. Jamie internally would feel rageful and helpless and would typically respond to her feeling of helplessness and "give up."

There are three levels of polarities in this example. Two levels are individual polarities of Jamie and Doug. Doug had a polarity along the lines of, "I love my wife and I value our partnership, but I'm afraid that she will leave me if I act wrongly." Jamie's polarity was something like, "I value dialogue with my husband and having his input, but I no longer want to try to involve him because I end up getting angry." The third polarity is at the couple system level: "We care about and love each other, but we can't stand *how* we are with each other." When these polarities show up in a sandtray scene and during the processing phase, *it matters not with which you begin the polarities process as I described in Chapter 4, because they are interrelated.* These polarities sustain each other and exist in parallel. However, I tend to lean toward identifying the individual polarities first when a couple creates individual trays, and then work with them to identify the core systems polarity. Now, imagine a family of five people with five individual polarities and a system polarity, and perhaps subsystem polarities. It is complex from a conceptual standpoint but keep it simple. Remember, HST is not about fixing problems or developing solutions.

Resistance is the second dynamic that will naturally emerge in couples and family HST. In couples work, Zinker (1994/1998) noted that "[r]esistance can occur within the couple at their contact boundary, or the couple may form a subsystem in resisting the therapist's intervention" (p. 186). Resistance patterns will be the same in either circumstance. If a couple tends to retroflect with each other, then they will retroflect with the therapist if they mount a defense in therapy. This dynamic becomes more complicated, of course, in family therapy where there are multiple subsystems, thus, multiple habits of resistance. Humanistic sandtray therapists approach resistance in systems therapy by *allowing the individual and the subsystem to have its defenses and using the process I outlined in Chapter 4*.

Conclusion

Although couples and family HST is more complex from a conceptual point of view and tends to be more action-oriented, the goals remain the same as in individual HST. HST allows therapists to use the power of creativity and metaphor to engage couples and families to discover themselves and reclaim a sense of a relational home. Considerations for humanistic sandtray therapists include modifying their sandtray collection, transitioning from individual to joint trays, providing sandtray prompts that bring to light relational strengths and vulnerabilities, maintaining facilitative responses designed to enhance awareness and highlight paradox, and attending to polarities and resistance.

References

Hays, P. A. (2022). *Addressing cultural complexities in counseling and clinical practice: An intersectional approach* (4th ed.). American Psychological Association. https://doi.org/10.1037/0000277-000

Homeyer, L. E., & Sweeney, D. S. (2023). *Sandtray therapy: A practical manual* (4th ed.). Routledge.

Satir, V. (1983). *Conjoint family therapy*. Science and Behavior Books.

Sweeney, D., & Rocha, S. (2000). Using play therapy to assess family dynamics. In R. Watts (Ed.), *Techniques in marriage and family counseling, Volume 1* (pp. 33–47). American Counseling Association.

Whitaker, C., & Keith, D. (1981). Symbolic-experiential therapy. In A. Gurman & D. Kniskern (Eds.), *Handbook of family therapy* (pp. 187–225). Brunner/Mazel.

Zinker, J. C. (1994/1998). *In search of good form: Gestalt therapy with couples and families*. Gestalt Institute of Cleveland Press.

Chapter 11

Humanistic Sandtray Therapy in School and Community Counseling Settings

Ryan D. Foster, Ryan Holliman, and Pedro J. Blanco

Access to mental health care varies widely across the United States. The number of people who are diagnosed with some form of mental illness and do not receive treatment is staggering; as of 2022, more than half of adults, or 27 million people, fit into this category, and 60 percent of young people under the age of 18 who were diagnosed with depression did not receive any mental health care services (Mental Health America, 2022). A number of causal factors have created this unfortunate scenario, and one, in particular, raises an alarm: 11.1 percent of people in the United States were uninsured, and 8.1 percent of minors who had insurance did not have mental health coverage as of 2022. These statistics are one reason that mental health providers can do a whole lot of good in two settings that are not fully dependent on insurance reimbursement and are increasingly on the front lines of equitable mental health services: schools and communities.

All three of us have worked in community mental health and school counseling settings providing play therapy and sandtray therapy, and we have also created and directed programs in which the goals were to integrate sandtray and play therapy with children, adolescents, and adults. Many of the clients with whom we have worked came from socioeconomically disadvantaged backgrounds. Most of the schools with which we have partnered were categorized as Title I, which are schools with a high percentage of low-income students. In one community counseling clinic, some of our clients paid $1 per session. We have seen the power of providing creative interventions in environments where the students and clients may not have any other option for mental health care. We have also seen notable change and growth take place with clients and students using sandtray. In this chapter, our aim is to provide you with guidance on establishing and maintaining an HST program in school and community counseling settings.

HST in School Counseling Settings

There is reason to believe that HST could be an important part of a school counseling program because of the dire need for children and adolescents

DOI: 10.4324/9781032664996-14

to have increased access to mental health services in schools. Of the public schools in the United States, 96 percent provided some kind of mental health service to students in their schools during the 2021–2022 school year (Institute of Education Sciences, 2022); 84 percent of mental health services in public schools consisted of individual counseling. However, 88 percent of public schools indicated that there were three primary obstacles to providing mental health services: not enough counseling staff to handle the number of students in need, not enough licensed mental health providers on staff, and not enough money. These obstacles are probably no surprise to those of you who are school counselors or school mental health therapists. Schools need creative solutions to the hurdles they face in addressing their kids' mental health needs. In this section, we will discuss why HST makes for a relevant part of a school counseling program, ways to convince stakeholders to devote resources to sandtray in schools, and practical approaches to setting up a sandtray collection.

Rationale for HST Programs in Schools

Most children who receive mental health counseling get it at school (Rock & Leff, 2015). Sallman (2007) noted several reasons that expressive therapies were a logical fit for school counseling environments. First, students are readily available and, as noted, are in high need of mental health services. Parents do not have to struggle with how to pay for counseling or how to provide regular transportation for their kids to get to a counselor. Relatedly, changes can be seen quite readily in the school environment by teachers and other school staff. Second, safety and trust in the therapeutic relationship can form quickly because of children's familiarity with the school counselor and environment. Therefore, the process of awareness and change in HST can move more swiftly, which is a good fit for understaffed school counseling environments. Third, there is an element of consistency by conducting HST in schools in terms of the environment, the counseling space, and the sandtray materials, allowing for significant depth of exploration of children's worlds and issues. Finally, humanistic sandtray therapists have access to consult with many significant people involved in children's lives, such as teachers, parents, and school administrators.

ASCA National Model Alignment

An important keystone of any program that therapists wish to integrate into a school counseling setting is alignment with the American School Counseling Association (ASCA) national model (2019). The national model establishes a framework for an overall program of school counseling and guidance services along with expected outcomes in students and an implementation process. We argue that HST is an intervention that fits well into the four major components of the ASCA national model: define, manage, deliver, and assess. Not only is this a conceptual argument, but also a practical one, as administrative stakeholders will want to know how an intervention like HST fits into the scope of a school counseling program. The *define* aspect of the model establishes the standards that a counseling program for a campus should follow. These program standards include professional standards for ethical and effective work as a school counselor and standards for child mindset and behavior. The mindsets that school counseling programs should instill in students include:

- Belief in the development of the whole self.
- Sense of acceptance, support, and inclusion for self and others at school.
- Positive attitude between work and learning.
- Self-confidence in ability to succeed.
- Belief in using ability to their fullest to achieve high-quality results and outcomes.
- Understanding that life-long learning is necessary for long-term success (ASCA, 2021, p. 2).

Also, there are 30 different behavioral standards grouped into three categories: learning strategies, self-management skills, and social skills (ASCA, 2019). HST is suited especially to the development of several of these mindsets and behavioral categories, making it an excellent choice for an intervention within a school counseling program. First, polarities work within HST allows for the recognition of different aspects of the client's self, which may range from physical, academic, mental, and social-emotional selves. These will be especially helpful in achieving the standards of "belief in the development of the whole self" and "sense of acceptance for others and self." Furthermore, HST helps emphasize capacities for perseverance, self-responsibility, and coping skills as the individual learns to gradually move toward the life-long journey of self-discovery and acceptance.

The *manage* domain of the ASCA national model (2019) refers to the ways in which a school counselor seeks to plan and focus the efforts of their school counseling program, which may include such activities as developing action plans, creating annual student outcome goals, gathering data from advisory councils, and more. When conducting the activities in the planning phase of the national model, there are several considerations that a school counselor must balance. One of the first concerns is that a school counselor's role is not typically directed toward long-term depth therapy models, and the ASCA model defines the role of a school counselor as involving *short-term counseling* as well as providing referrals to *long-term support*. A recent meta-analysis on sand-based interventions by Wiersma et al. (2022) found that participants could receive clinical benefits in as few as ten sessions, indicating that it meets some of the unique challenges of a school setting. Another consideration is the broad range of mental health issues that a school counseling program must address. School counselors may address such varied issues as mood disorders, trauma, addictions, grief, anxiety disorders, suicidal ideation, and many more mental health challenges. Thus, when school counselors choose interventions, it behooves them to select one that can be adaptable to a wide range of needs. HST has a broad range of applications that can address psychological dynamics that underlie many disorders. Furthermore, HST can be integrated as a part of an overall therapy relationship, making it adaptable. Finally, school counselors must consider a range of developmental levels. Counselors at elementary schools, middle schools/junior high schools, and high schools have a broad range of students that can vary within grade levels across the developmental continuum in regard to emotional, cognitive, and interpersonal presentations. Not only is there a vast array of differences from students in sixth grade to seniors in high school, but it is widely known that a student's developmental level does not always equal their chronological age. Sandtray is an especially versatile tool because of its adaptability for various developmental levels. Due to the nature of HST, the amount of verbalization can vary, with some students having the option to focus on the tray itself for much of the session, and other students using the tray as a tool to explore issues in depth with more abstract discussions of psychological dynamics. For these reasons, HST is a well-suited intervention for schools.

The *deliver* domain is composed of two kinds of activities: direct and indirect services (ASCA, 2019). Direct services are those provided to students to meet their counseling needs, such as individual or group counseling. Indirect services benefit students but tend to comprise support functions such as consultation with other professionals in school, collaborative initiatives within the community, and referral to external providers. HST is an obviously appropriate intervention for direct services and, in addition to the more traditional individual HST model, there have been research studies indicating efficacy of group sandtray experiences in schools (Flahive & Ray, 2007; Shen & Armstrong, 2008).

Finally, for the *assess* domain, school counselors evaluate the overall impact of the program, which may answer such questions as who participated in school counseling activities, what ASCA (2019) mindsets and behaviors the students developed, and how school counseling activities impacted student attendance, discipline, and/or academic achievement. HST can provide a beneficial tool for the assess domain. Although, obviously, measuring who participated and the impacts of HST on discipline, academic achievement, and attendance are more quantitative measurements, using HST can be a helpful assessment tool to measure changes in mindset. As discussed previously, a common prompt in HST is to ask a participant to create their world in the sand tray. Through a qualitative analysis, a counselor can assess changes in mindsets that occur over the course of extended HST as well as using a single sandtray to evaluate potential mindsets and behaviors that have been instilled in the child. For example, imagine a child who may be dealing with socialization issues and is provided HST as an intervention. At the beginning of the work, they might create a sandtray in which one human figure is isolated from a large group of figures by a moat; during processing, they may share the feeling of being isolated and the thought that they do not fit into any of the groups at their school. However, during HST sessions further along in counseling, the student might create a tray in which they have made a bridge that reaches across the moat, and they may share feeling more connected with their peers and having more confidence in their ability to make friends. By a qualitative analysis of themes in HST in this case, the student has developed behavior B-SS 2, "Positive, respectful and supportive relationships with students who are similar to and different from them" (ASCA, 2021, p. 2), which is one of the listed behaviors for student success in the ASCA national model. In addition, individual sandtrays done with children at one point in time can give insights into where children may have demonstrated gains in mindsets and behaviors for success. By combining both quantitative and qualitative data, school counselors and other mental health professionals in schools can observe a more accurate picture of the mental health of a school population, and sandtrays can provide a much-needed qualitative aspect to said data.

Convincing School Stakeholders

Providing HST in schools requires a persuasion effort on the part of mental health professionals. Unfortunately, therapists often convince themselves that they are no good at this kind of thing. However, we agree with Yalom's (1980) contention that therapy at its very foundation is an attempt to persuade. Thus, we encourage you to approach boldly the task of gaining the support of district and school administrators, teachers, parents, and, if you are an outside mental health therapist, school counselors, by remembering that many of the key tasks in such an undertaking are well within your skillset as a therapist.

The first step that we recommend starts with *perspective taking*. It can be easy for therapists to get entrenched in their own perspectives and viewpoints. For example, as a therapist you might view the idea of sandtray as important and beneficial to students because of its potential to help students identify and work through key mental health dynamics. However, you must remember when advocating for an HST program to a principal that although mental health is certainly good to promote, the key mission of the school is to provide education to students and bolster future academic success. It can be easy to forget that in schools, mental health is not an end unto itself, but rather a pathway to the ultimate goal of removing barriers to educational attainment. So, in discussing HST with a school administrator such as a principal, you might emphasize the power of HST to help students address mental health issues such as anxiety and depression, which might otherwise impede a student's ability to attend to lesson plans in class or complete assignments to acquire academic competencies.

The second step in convincing school stakeholders is *preparation*. You should prepare formal report and presentation materials that use language accessible by each stakeholder group. Include elements of the rationale for HST programs that we outlined earlier in this chapter. Create an "elevator speech" that addresses common concerns of stakeholders. We discuss our suggestions for responding to these concerns later in this chapter.

The third step is *initiating contact*. Initiating an HST program in a school begins with the first contact with the lead school counseling administrator. In some states and in charter school systems, these lead administrators are at the district or system level. In other states or in private school environments, the first contact may be at the school where you plan to start a program. If you are a school counselor, our guess is that you already know who you would need to contact, and you may have enough independence that you can get the green light from your principal. The point here is, start at the top—whatever that means for you.

When meeting with administrative stakeholders, it is important that you emphasize that HST is a type of counseling that is appropriate for most kids aged 10 and up. Blalock (2023), echoing Homeyer and Sweeney (2023), recommended use of the term sandtray *counseling* rather than *therapy* because school stakeholders and even parents may be uncomfortable with the idea of therapy. Additionally, ensure that you provide administrative stakeholders with resources supporting the use of HST, including previous research (see Chapter 14) and your evaluation plans. Evaluation plans should include a method you will use to measure progress in the children to whom you provide HST. For example, you may use teacher reports, and both an informal and a formal quantitative measure such as the Achenbach System of Empirically Based Assessment (ASEBA; Achenbach, 2009) Teacher's Report Form (TRF). You might also use student grades, standardized academic achievement testing results, discipline referral data, or even problem-specific inventories such as the Children's Depression Inventory-2 (CDI-2; Kovacs, 2011) or the ASEBA Youth

Self-Report (YSR; Achenbach, 2009) to measure decreases in behavioral problems or improvement in affective symptoms that might be interfering with learning (Ray, 2011).

The third step is *meeting with school personnel*, which includes teachers, potentially school counselors, school administrators, and other staff. You could meet with them during staff development days or individually. Each school has its idiosyncratic expectations, and it is important to use active listening when meeting with personnel. When talking to teachers about HST, present the rationale and definition of sandtray and HST, procedures for referral, and a detailed walkthrough of the process. Educate them on the empirical support and implications for student learning and in-class behavior in order to promote the utility of HST. Understand that for teachers, the primary goal is learning, not necessarily mental health. Therefore, discussions should focus on ways that HST can enhance academic achievement and reduce barriers to learning. In addition, discuss the potential role of HST in reducing teacher stress due to decreased problematic in-class behaviors that lead to classroom distractions. The goal during these conversations should be to alleviate concerns and persuade school personnel that having an HST program at their school is designed to have a positive impact.

Addressing Stakeholder Concerns

Parents, teachers, and administrators will inevitably have concerns about how an HST program may negatively impact students, classroom functioning, and learning. We have found that these concerns tend to fall into two major categories: pull-out services issues and confidentiality concerns. In our experience, pull-out services issues tend to focus on two questions:

1. How much instructional time will this student miss? What will the impact be on the classroom when the counselor picks the child up and returns them?
2. What kind of stigma will this student face for going to counseling?

These are noteworthy questions to address. For missing class time, be honest about how long you plan for each HST session to last as well as how many times per week. One of us (Ryan Foster) directed an HST program in a middle school and, over the course of the semester, teachers began to express concerns about students missing time in core classes attached to areas on the state standardized tests. I adjusted the HST schedule so that students were only pulled from electives. Then, the electives teachers began to request that I not pull out their students from those classes. Eventually, I had to discuss the situation with the school counselor, and she was able to conduct a conversation with all the teachers. We found a solution in which students would be pulled toward the end of one class and returned to the following class. This move also decreased disrupting the same class twice in one period.

In terms of the potential for stigmatized counseling for students, we have found that this concern has decreased significantly among students themselves as contemporarily, the importance of mental health seems to have landed generationally. In fact, a middle school counselor with whom I (Ryan Foster) worked reported to me that students who did not qualify for our HST program requested to be put on a sandtray waitlist just in case an opportunity opened! In our experience, stigma emanates primarily from parents. We have worked in schools in communities where counseling and psychotherapy were seen as a threat to family boundaries. Our approach is to reach out to parents when they express a concern, actively listen, and, if parents remain unconvinced, to respect their points of view.

Inevitably, when beginning and maintaining an HST program in school, you will face concerns about confidentiality. If you are an outside therapist and not the school counselor, then often school personnel themselves will have questions about how documentation may be handled. These are the three most common questions we run into:

1. Are notes part of the educational record?
2. What to discuss with teachers/parents/principals?
3. How to communicate what is needed while still maintaining a sense of privacy for the child?

In terms of notes and how they are protected, it is typical for clinical notes to be excluded from educational records. You should outline this circumstance explicitly in informed consent forms. Often, we have found that school personnel are relieved by this response. The second question has come up for us in the main school office, hallways, or classrooms when principals or teachers check in with us. You should be prepared to give a vague response that respects the confidentiality of the student. Some principals will ask about specific students, particularly if it is a student who has a litany of office referrals. Principals have the right to know that a particular student is being seen for HST. You may want to discuss that the student is engaged in the process and appears to be benefiting, and follow up with your own inquiry—something like, "What have you noticed about Sarah since she has been in the HST program?" Parents may have more specific questions, and we recommend that you answer them in ways that respect the child's safety and trust in the therapeutic relationship. For example, sharing themes in their tray rather than describing the specific scene they created is one way to balance a parent's right to know how their kid is benefiting and the child's right to confidentiality.

Organizing a School-based HST Program

There are practical realities involved when organizing a school-based HST program. The major considerations we encourage you to attend to are time, space, and money. We favor discussing these issues with your school stakeholders. First is the issue of *time*. Session times in schools are different necessarily from a clinical setting. We recommend conducting 30-minute sandtray sessions. In our experience running HST programs in middle schools, half an hour is plenty of time to conduct an HST session from creation phase to processing phase.

The second issue is *money*. As discussed in previous chapters, getting a sandtray collection going can be costly. However, there are some avenues that may help lighten your financial load. Look for potential donations from businesses in the area that have supported your school in the past. Remember that many miniatures in your sandtray therapy collection need not be expensive or fancy. Discount stores often carry fairly inexpensive miniatures. Blalock (2023) provided other relevant suggestions in this area. She suggested enlisting the help of people in the therapist's or school counselor's social network to donate items like "fast food children's meal toys, old jewelry, used cake decorations, holiday decorations, small toys … dice, colored stones, and objects from board games" (p. 20).

The third issue is *space*. Depending on the size of your sandtray miniatures collection and your tray itself, HST can be conducted anywhere from a full-sized room to a storage closet. We have even occupied a corner of a classroom that was used for various programs like occupational and speech therapies. In these kinds of circumstances, it is easy to use your sandtray shelves to act as the "walls" of the corner of the room. When sharing a room, ensure that you can use the space uninterrupted due to confidentiality. We have worked in small spaces even with standard-sized sand trays wherein we were able to fit the tray, shelves, figurines, and two chairs.

Managing Your HST Program

Once stakeholders have approved your HST program, you will need to work to organize it. Ray (2011) created an eight-step model for establishing school-based CCPT programs, which we have adapted for HST programs. Step one is to calculate the number of available sandtray sessions that you have over the course of an academic semester. Your calculations should include the number of sandtray sessions that each child will receive, how long each session will last, how much time you will build in for returning each child to class, cleaning up the sandtray scene, pulling the next child out of class, and availability of the space in which you will be providing HST.

In addition, you should consider any school holidays or staff development days. When we oversee HST programs in middle schools, our calculations typically include six sessions of 30 minutes each per child, meeting once per week, building in ten minutes between each sandtray session to give time to return kids to class, clean up, and pick up the next child for their session.

The next step is to develop a referral list from parents, teachers, school counselors, and other school staff (Ray, 2011). When we have reached out to parents, we typically create a packet consisting of information about the HST program, a consent form, and any baseline measures that require parental input. We then work with the school counselor to place these packets in students' folders for them to take home. As you probably know, some of these packets make it home to parents or caregivers, and sometimes they do not!

Step three is to collect child background information (Ray, 2011). If you are the school counselor, you may already have some of this information available to you. Outside mental health therapists may need to develop a form to collect this information from school counselors, teachers, and parents. Background information should include demographics such as age, date of birth, racial and ethnic identity, gender identity, a brief mental health history, and any data that you intend to use as qualifiers for inclusion in your HST program. Example qualifiers may include academic achievement scores, the number of office referrals, a history of classroom behavioral disruptions, and other measures that are meant to establish baseline indicators such as the TRF.

Steps four and five involve analyzing the background information you have collected on each child to determine if their needs would be served better by referral to another program offered by the school district or an outside mental health provider (Ray, 2011). If a student has had a recent mental health crisis, they may not be a good fit for HST until they have stabilized. Once you have created a pool of potential HST program participants, step five is to rank children in order of need based on severity, particularly as it relates to being at risk for school failure based on poor academic achievement or behavioral issues. Once you have completed these tasks, then you should have a final list of children who you plan to invite to participate in your HST program.

Step six is to create a schedule of HST sandtray sessions (Ray, 2011). Your program may consist of individual HST, group HST, or both. In the case of offering both individual and group HST, part of step six should be to determine which sandtray format would best meet each child's needs. For those children who struggle with socialization, peer relationships, or a sense of belonging, group HST may be an excellent fit. Individual HST may fit best for children whose struggles are related to issues such as depression, anxiety, trauma, or family conflict. Once you have created a schedule for students included in your HST programs, then comes the action phase. The first time you meet with a student, you should concentrate on establishing a therapeutic relationship. In addition, you may be gathering baseline measurements for the indicators you intend on measuring if you are using mental health instruments such as the CDI-2 or the YSR, which require children to self-report.

Once children have completed their HST sessions, step seven is to reassess them for progress (Ray, 2011) using the measurements that you gathered at baseline, such as academic achievement scores, teacher reports, or mental health questionnaires. You will need to quickly analyze these data to complete step eight, which is to determine if children in your HST program have made progress. If they have made progress based on standards that you have determined, then terminate them from the HST program and provide any needed referrals. For children who have not demonstrated progress, attempt to schedule them for additional sandtray sessions.

HST in Community Counseling Settings

When I (Ryan Foster) was looking to apply to graduate programs in counseling, I came across the term community counseling. It became my specialization during my master's counseling program and my first class was titled as such. My eyes were opened to the history of the community counseling movement and how it appears in modern-day counseling settings. From that first semester of graduate school onward, the concept of community counseling has been the lens through which I view my roles as a mental health counselor, supervisor, and counselor educator. Lewis et al. (2011) defined community counseling as "a comprehensive helping framework that is grounded in multicultural competence and oriented toward social justice" (p. 9). Commonly, community counseling services take place in agencies, a broad term encompassing public and private, for-profit (including profit with purpose) and non-profit, organizations (Corey, Corey, & Corey, 2024). We believe that HST is a community counseling direct service intervention that can expose clients from diverse backgrounds to acceptance, growth, healing, and connection. In this section, we will focus on practical issues for consideration in community agency settings such as stakeholder inclusion, funding, space, and training for clinicians who use sandtray. We will also provide guidance regarding documentation best practices.

Community Counseling Agency Organizational Considerations

Sandtray therapy can sometimes appear nearly impossible to integrate into a community agency setting. Like schools, agencies have limited funding and space, and practitioners who work in agencies have the Sisyphean task of convincing stakeholders that creative interventions, especially those that do not emanate from cognitive-behavioral therapy, fit in settings that demand accountability and program evaluation. Astramovich and Coker (2007) defined accountability as "providing specific information to stakeholders and other supervising authorities about the effectiveness and efficiency of counseling services" (p. 163) and argued that program evaluation was a precursor to accountability. They noted that counselors should build in program evaluation practices to "plan, implement, and refine counseling practice regardless of the need to demonstrate accountability" (p. 163). Essentially, accountability legitimizes to others the value of the therapist's work. Evidence-based creative approaches to counseling, such as child-centered play therapy and Adlerian play therapy (Association for Play Therapy, n.d.), have paved the way for humanistic sandtray therapists to begin building HST programs in community agency settings. Major organizational considerations worth noting when building an HST program in a community counseling agency are stakeholder inclusion, funding, space, and practitioner training.

Stakeholders

Community counseling agency stakeholders go beyond the walls of the practice space. They stretch deep into the community and include any person or institution who may be impacted by the agency's services (Boulmetis & Dutwin, 2000). Therefore, when you design an HST program for your agency, you must consider including the wider community and leaders from local organizations when gathering feedback and communicating program evaluation outcomes (Astramovich & Coker, 2007). For example, you may want to include leaders from local religious institutions and social service agencies, school counselors, and parents. When designing an accountability plan, establish timeframes for reporting back to stakeholders in a jargon-free format and in a way that honors their relationship to the agency.

Funding

Identifying funding sources for programs that include creative interventions like HST can be challenging; however, what we have found is that many sources care more about the outcome than how to get there, as long as there is a good rationale for an efficient program. HST can be an efficient intervention because of its depth-oriented focus—sandtray therapy can jump-start client healing. Humanistic sandtray therapists focus on awareness rather than specific symptoms, and because HST is flexible in terms of format (individual, group, couples, and family therapy) and adaptable across spectrums of diverse identities, it can be a cost-effective way of treatment.

When applying for funding, most of the budget will be marked for the sandtray collection and practitioner training, adding to its cost effectiveness.

Space

Space is an ongoing issue at many community counseling agencies. Therapists must share consultation rooms often, furniture is donated commonly, and there may be little room for specialized equipment like a sand tray and shelving set aside for miniatures. However, there are ways to take advantage of existing spaces to make room for a sandtray collection. One option is to keep trays and miniatures in a storage space and get them out when you plan to use them with a client. Additionally, if there is a dedicated play therapy room at your agency, you could use part of a wall for shelving and a sandtray.

Training

Of significant importance is the issue of ensuring that more than one clinician at your agency is trained in HST (see Chapter 12). It would be very difficult to convince stakeholders, funding sources, and agency administrators in charge of programming available physical spaces of the potential value of an HST program if only one therapist is qualified to provide these services. Therefore, it would be of significant value to identify clinicians who practice from a humanistic point of view or have experience in CCPT.

Documentation of HST Sessions

Documentation is perhaps one of the least favorite activities for which therapists are responsible, and we must say, it is not that fun about which to write, either! However, it is more than a "necessary evil" in psychotherapy; we consider it a deeply intimate practice that can act as a benefit to client care. When we write progress notes or revisit our informed consent forms, we think about the person behind the label of "client" with whom we work. Therefore, we encourage you to approach your clinical documentation in HST as a valuable part of how humanistic sandtray therapists invite clients into their healing process. In this section, we will discuss how to approach documenting HST sessions in progress notes as well as how to form language around HST in your informed consent form.

Progress Notes

Progress notes are an ethical and legal requirement of mental health practitioners (Corey et al., 2024). Good clinical documentation can also assist you in conceptualization and informal assessment by allowing you to see the progression of a client's sandtrays over time. Most practitioners use a telehealth platform to record digital progress notes. Some community agencies have created their own format and others use widely adapted formats such as SOAP (subjective, objective, assessment, plan) or DAP (data, assessment, plan) notes. Similar to interventions such as child-centered play therapy (Ray, 2011), when documenting HST sessions, therapists should capture a holistic summary of the session without interpreting elements of the process that are unclear.

There is a template for HST progress notes in Appendix A that you are welcome to use as is or adapt to existing documentation formats of your practice. It is based on the DAP note format. The *data* section is where therapists note concrete observations such as client affect, mood, general themes of what they discussed, and any interventions that the therapist used. In the *assessment* section, therapists document their conceptualization in terms of client progress, how they are responding to the treatment plan, a summary of results of any assessment instruments used, and the client's diagnosis. The assessment section should relate to information in the data section. The *plan* section includes when and where the next session will take place, any referrals that the therapist gave the client, and any modifications to the client's treatment plan that the therapist recommends based on information from data and assessment.

If you are unable to use the template provided in Appendix A, we recommend that you include similar elements in progress notes that document an HST session. Although the plan section does not differ significantly from a standard progress note that you use for non-HST sessions, there are areas we recommend you describe in the data and assessment sections of a progress note. In the data section, at a minimum, we advise you to include:

- Client's affect and mood.
- Safety concerns (e.g., suicidal or homicidal ideation).
- The sandtray prompt that you used.
- HST interventions used (e.g., reflections, centering exercise, immediacy, guiding into–staying with–going deeper into emotions, enactment, polarities work).
- Categories of sandtray miniatures that the client used.
- A digital photo of the sandtray scene.

In the assessment section, we recommend you include conceptualization regarding:

- Disposition of the therapeutic relationship and how it impacted the session.
- Any polarities that you identified and/or explored with the client.
- A summary of metaphors in the tray.

- Any contact disturbances that emerged.
- A summary of your overall conceptualization and client progress.

Informed Consent

Informed consent is both a document and a process (Corey et al., 2024). Although informed consent is a legal and ethical responsibility of therapists, it is part of good clinical care, too (Wheeler & Bertram, 2019). We highly recommend that you provide a specific informed consent form and process for HST. HST informed consent can be provided either as an integration into your existing informed consent document, or as a separate document. Therapists who work in agency settings may be disallowed to change the informed consent document that clinicians use and, if this is the case for you, hopefully you are able to work with your agency to provide a separate sandtray informed consent form for your clients. See Appendix B for a template that you can use. If you want to create your own, we recommend that you include, at a minimum, the following in your sandtray informed consent:

- Professional qualifications and background as they pertain to sandtray therapy.
- Risks and benefits of engaging in sandtray therapy.
- The voluntary nature of sandtray therapy.
- Language informing your clients that you will take photographs of their sandtrays and that these photographs will become part of their clinical files.

One way that we like to incorporate informed consent as a process into our sandtray work, particularly when sandtray is brand new to clients, is to add language to the prompts we use. We might add something like, "What you choose to share is up to you." Using this statement encourages client autonomy, which is a significant part of safety and trust.

Conclusion

There is an incredibly high need for dependable access to mental health care in the United States and across the world. In the United States, schools and community agencies are at the frontlines of providing mental health services for children, adolescents, and adults, and we encourage therapists and school counselors who work in these settings to bring sandtray therapy to the clients they serve. Creative interventions like HST can be a valuable way of providing powerfully therapeutic, efficient, and cost-effective care to clients who seek healing and growth.

References

Achenbach, T. M. (2009). *The Achenbach System of Empirically Based Assessment (ASEBA): Development, findings, theory, and applications.* University of Vermont Research Center for Children, Youth, & Families.

American School Counselor Association (ASCA). (2019). *The ASCA national model: A framework for school counseling programs* (4th ed.). Author.

American School Counselor Association (ASCA). (2021). ASCA student standards: Mindsets and behaviors for student success. Author. https://www.schoolco unselor.org/getmedia/7428a787-a452-4abb-afec-d78ec77870cd/Mindsets-Behaviors.pdf

Association for Play Therapy. (n.d.). Research and practice. https://www.a4pt.org/page/Research

Astramovich, R. L., & Coker, J. K. (2007). Program evaluation: The accountability bridge model for counselors. *Journal of Counseling & Development, 85*(2), 131–255. https://doi.org/10.1002/j.1556-6678.2007.tb00459.x

Blalock, S. M. (2023). School-based sandtray counseling on a shoe string. *Journal of Creativity in Mental Health, 18*(1), 16–27. https://doi.org/10.1080/15401383.2021.1928575

Boulmetis, J., & Dutwin, P. (2000). *The ABCs of evaluation: Timeless techniques for program and project managers.* Jossey-Bass.

Corey, G., Corey, M. S., & Corey, C. (2024). *Issues and ethics in the helping professions* (11th ed.). Cengage Learning.

Flahive, M. H. W., & Ray, D. (2007). Effect of group sandtray therapy with preadolescents. *The Journal for Specialists in Group Work, 32*(4), 362–382. https://doi.org/10.1080/01933920701476706

Homeyer, L. E., & Sweeney, D. S. (2023). *Sandtray therapy: A practical manual* (4th ed.). Routledge. https://doi.org/10.4324/9781003221418

Institute of Education Sciences. (2022). *Mental health and well-being of students and staff during the pandemic.* https://ies.ed.gov/schoolsurvey/spp/SPP_April_Infographic_Mental_Health_and_Well_Being.pdf

Kovacs, M., & MHS Staff. (2011). *Children's Depression Inventory 2nd Edition (CDI 2). Technical manual.* Multi-Health Systems.

Lewis, J. A., Lewish, M. D., Daniels, J. A., & D'Andrea, M. J. (2011). *Community counseling: A multicultural-social justice perspective* (4th ed.). Brooks/Cole, Cengage Learning.

Mental Health America. (2022). *The state of mental health in America.* https://mhanational.org/sites/default/files/2022%20State%20of%20Mental%20Health%20in%20America.pdf

Ray, D. C. (2011). *Advanced play therapy: Essential conditions, knowledge, and skills for child practice.* Routledge.

Rock, E., & Leff, E. H. (2015). The professional school counselor and students with disabilities. In B. T. Erford (Ed.), *Transforming the school counseling profession* (4th ed., pp. 350–391). Pearson.

Sallman, C. M. (2007). Play therapy: An overview and marketing plan. [Unpublished master's thesis]. Kansas State University.

Shen, Y. P., & Armstrong, S. A. (2008). Impact of group sandtray therapy on the self-esteem of young adolescent girls. *The Journal for Specialists in Group Work*, *33*(2), 118–137. https://doi.org/10.1080/01933920801977397

Wheeler, A. M., & Bertram, B. (2019). *The counselor and the law: A guide to legal and ethical practice* (8th ed.). American Counseling Association.

Wiersma, J. K., Freedle, L. R., McRoberts, R., & Solberg, K. B. (2022). A meta-analysis of sandplay therapy treatment outcomes. *International Journal of Play Therapy*, *31*(4), 197–215. https://doi.org/10.1037/pla0000180

Yalom, I. D. (1980). *Existential psychotherapy*. Basic Books.

Part IV

Training, Supervision, and Research

Chapter 12

Humanistic Sandtray Therapy Group Training Model

When I first learned about sandtray therapy as a master's student at Texas State University, my professor, Dr. Linda Homeyer, emphasized an experiential approach to our learning. I do not remember how many sandtrays my classmates and I did, but I remember there were a lot of them! Subsequently, when I was trained by Dr. Steve Armstrong in his humanistic approach to sandtray therapy, it was almost entirely experiential. Learning by doing fits rather nicely with humanistic therapists' view of how people learn and change. Sandtray experts (Armstrong, 2008; Homeyer & Lyles, 2022; Homeyer & Sweeney, 2023) have emphasized that there really is no better or more effective way to learn sandtray than by doing sandtrays, observing others process sandtrays, and discussing learnings in group settings. If you want to develop sound skills in HST, you must commit yourself to engaging with vulnerability and openness to experiential modes of learning sandtray. Thus, in this chapter, I will discuss the HST group training model that I employ, developed originally by Dr. Steve Armstrong.

At this point in the book, you may be interested in practicing sandtray therapy if you have not before or honing your practice if you have been doing it for a while. There is a growing number of formal training opportunities through various institutes and organizations in both sandtray and sandplay therapy around the globe. If you want to practice sandtray therapy, you should seek out formal advanced training. Reading this book is an excellent start, and experiential training is what will really solidify your skills and approach. I would never recommend that a therapist practice sandtray therapy without formal experiential training.

If you are interested in becoming a humanistic sandtray therapist as described in this book, the only place at which training is offered currently in this model is through the Humanistic Sandtray Therapy Institute (HSTI). I founded the HSTI in 2023 after my mentor, Steve Armstrong, died, to continue training practitioners in this model. If you decide to train at HSTI, you can choose to meet additional requirements to obtain your certification as a Certified Humanistic Sandtray Therapist (CHST). Not everyone

DOI: 10.4324/9781032664996-16

who participates in my trainings goes on to become CHSTs. However, enrolling in the certification route supports your growth of skills and ability to theoretically conceptualize clients because of the intensive supervision requirements. If you have interest, you can visit my website and learn more at https://humanisticsandtray.com.

Examples of HST Sessions

I have made example videos of HST sessions with a variety of populations on the HSTI website at https://humanisticsandtray.com/videos. Many of the populations about which you have read in this book have an example video. These are not roleplay videos; these are real people with genuine areas of their worlds that they explore in their trays. They are designed to pair with the content in this book.

Prerequisites of HST Training

Before you seek training in HST, Armstrong (2008) recommended that therapists have professional experience with child-centered play therapy (CCPT). I echo Armstrong's sentiment for therapists who work with older children and preadolescents. The skills that therapists learn when training in and practicing CCPT complement HST very well. Skills like observation of non-verbals, reflection of feeling, and staying in the metaphor are essential to the practice of CCPT (Ray, 2011) and mirror basic skills of HST, too. Conversely, I have trained many therapists who have little to no background in CCPT and they have become excellent humanistic sandtray therapists; however, these trainees typically work with older adolescents and adults. I believe so strongly in humanistic sandtray therapists who work with children and preadolescents having a background in CCPT that I only endorse them when they receive formal training in both approaches.

Another prerequisite of HST is that you align with humanistic philosophy. I also think contemporary psychodynamic approaches fit well with HST because of their emphasis on the here and now. However, it would be very difficult to integrate HST if you practice from a cognitive-behavioral point of view because of key philosophical and theoretical differences. Our emphasis on emotions as precursors to thoughts and behaviors separates the HST philosophy from cognitive approaches in which thoughts are a precursor. Nevertheless, I have trained practitioners from cognitive and reality therapy backgrounds who have changed their belief systems to be more in line with HST, and this has benefited their sandtray work with clients because they discovered truths about themselves and who they were in the midst of training. As I think about these experiences, I feel a deep sense of meaning because I witnessed these clinicians' increased awareness processes and a real shift into more congruence and authenticity.

Core Training in HST

The core training in HST consists of a Level I and a Level II program. I have trained clinicians across the United States, with most of my trainings taking place in the Dallas/Fort Worth metroplex. However, I have traveled to other regions of the country for these trainings. I train small groups of six to eight clinicians. Trainees learn basic sandtray concepts and practices as well as HST-specific attitudes and skills such as facilitative responses, engaging in the here and now, person-centered and gestalt principles, levels of processing within metaphors, the entering into–staying with–going deeper into emotional experiencing cycle, polarities work, and working with resistance. Table 12.1 summarizes the goals for participants in each level of training.

Table 12.1 Training goals of HSTI Levels I and II

Level I	Level II
• Learn the basics of sandtray including conducting a session, determining clients appropriate for the modality, understanding of rationale for sandtray, and practical matters such as acquisition of miniatures. • Become more proficient at understanding and practicing humanistic sandtray processing through live demonstrations, experiential activities, and group discussion. • Improve ability to respond to non-verbal, here-and-now expressions of emotion, work effectively in the here and now, see and respond to polarities, and facilitate awareness and depth of experiencing. • Enhance self-awareness, experience emotion in the moment, and gain insight into personal issues that may hinder client growth if not addressed. • Receive supervision and feedback during group sandtray experiences and observations.	• Continue to develop ability to respond to non-verbal expressions of emotion in sandtray, work effectively in the here and now, see and respond to polarities, and facilitate awareness and depth of experiencing. • Enhance self-awareness, experience emotion in the moment, and gain insight into personal issues that may hinder client growth if not addressed. • Learn how to gently guide sandtray clients to a deeper level of experiencing. • Demonstrate the ability to utilize a descriptive mode of responding that helps clients to explore emotions and avoid analysis and explanations of inner experiencing. • Learn to recognize, identify, separate, and work effectively with both sides of polarities. • Learn the humanistic approach to working with resistance including the following: Recognizing physical blocks and responding in ways that help the client feel safer; gently guiding clients through a process of awareness of their defenses in the here and now; and helping clients to utilize ways of their defenses increasing tension before relaxing such as accentuating the obvious.

Some clinicians who attend trainings are well-seasoned therapists with years of professional experience; some are graduate students working on their degrees in mental health therapy; and others are somewhere in between those states. Each level of training lasts for two and a half days. They are intensive and almost entirely experiential in nature. Trainees work in pairs or triads and practice sandtray skills that they have learned. There are some didactic components, of course, yet there is a heavy focus on train-ees observing me work with them within the small group to practice the intricacies of the HST approach. Trainees create their own sandtrays and have numerous opportunities to practice, observe, process, and discuss. I have witnessed meaningful shifts in trainees who attend these trainings, both personally and professionally.

If you recall my discussion in Chapter 1 on qualities of effective human-istic sandtray therapists, you may remember my emphasis on the correl-ation between personal and professional ways of being. Side effects of HST training often include increased awareness of this connection. HST training requires trainees to be open to exploring self and person of the sandtray therapist (Homeyer & Lyles, 2022). One of the most impactful ways in which I work with trainees is by practicing here-and-now awareness and inviting them to begin to establish this way of being as a safe place to which to return.

Certification

There is an increasing number of professional credentials in sandtray and sandplay therapy. Credentials communicate to clients and other professionals that therapists have training and professional experience in their specializa-tion. The Humanistic Sandtray Therapy Institute offers both a certification as a Certified Humanistic Sandtray Therapist (CHST) and opportunities to become a CHST-Supervisor. In order to qualify as a CHST, therapists must complete successfully the HSTI Level I and Level II trainings and attend several individual supervision sessions with a CHST-Supervisor. Therapists who participate in the certification route are required to create several of their own sandtrays during supervision. In addition, therapists must video record their sandtray sessions with their clients so that they can receive feed-back on their developing HST skills from their supervisors. I discuss more about HST supervision in Chapter 13. If you are interested in becoming a CHST, then you may visit my website at https://humanisticsandtray.com.

Expanded HST Training

The core training in HST is only the beginning of your journey. Even after becoming fully certified as a CHST, humanistic sandtray therapists best serve their clients by continuing to develop their approach to sandtray therapy. If humanistic sandtray therapists intend to work with groups, couples, or families, then they must seek further training opportunities to gain competence in working in these therapy situations. HSTI offers expanded training opportunities both in-person and digitally so that you can hone your approach and continue to develop your skillsets.

Conclusion

It is not good enough to read a book or attend a one-hour workshop on sandtray therapy in order to utilize this approach with clients. Therapists who want to become trained in HST can attend intensive experiential trainings at the Humanistic Sandtray Therapy Institute, which offers several opportunities to learn and gain experience in HST. Becoming a skillful and experienced humanistic sandtray therapist requires a dedication to increasing awareness and lifelong personal and professional development.

References

Armstrong, S. A. (2008). *Sandtray therapy: A humanistic approach*. Ludic Press.

Homeyer, L. E., & Lyles, M. N. (2022). *Advanced sandtray therapy: Digging deeper into clinical practice*. Routledge. https://doi.org/10.4324/9781003095491

Homeyer, L. E., & Sweeney, D. S. (2023). *Sandtray therapy: A practical manual* (4th ed.). Routledge. https://doi.org/10.4324/9781003221418

Ray, D. C. (2011). *Advanced play therapy: Essential conditions, knowledge, and skills for child practice*. Routledge.

Chapter 13

Humanistic Sandtray Supervision

Supervision is a flagstone process that instigates and supports growth as a professional mental health therapist. Although supervision has a lot in common with counseling and psychotherapy, it is a distinct professional role (Bernard & Goodyear, 2019). Clinicians-in-training encounter supervision first during graduate school, continue into post-graduate and pre-licensure experiences, and may return to it when seeking additional graduate degrees, post-licensure certifications, or licenses. Although one of the major goals of supervision is to ensure that supervisees become excellent clinicians, supervision acts also as a gatekeeper to keep bad actors from becoming independently licensed practitioners. Ultimately, good supervision is designed to ensure client welfare. And good supervision provides supervisees with opportunities to increase their awareness of self and other (Bernard, 1979, 1997; Kagan & Kagan, 1997; Loganbill, Hardy, & Delworth, 1982; Rønnestad & Skovholt, 2003; Stoltenberg, McNeill, & Delworth, 1998).

Creative approaches have quite a bit of utility in supervision. Newsome, Henderson, and Veach (2011) noted that expressive arts can provoke access to supervisees' intuition, inner experiencing, and "help supervisees expand their awareness of self and others" (p. 145). Casado-Kehoe and Ybañez-Llorente (2018) similarly stated that using expressive arts in supervision from a gestalt orientation can model effective clinical practice, client conceptualization, and self-awareness. Perryman and Anderson (2011) and Perryman, Moss, and Anderson (2016) described their use of sandtray in supervision based on a combined model incorporating the discrimination model (Bernard, 1979, 1997), the integrated developmental model (IDM; Stoltenberg et al., 1998), and person-centered and gestalt theory. They drew on characteristics of person-centered supervision relationships to establish a safe foundation in which supervisees could explore self as therapist and work within the metaphor of the tray, activating supervisory foci inherent to the IDM. Perryman et al. (2021) reported

DOI: 10.4324/9781032664996-17

results of a qualitative study of their model with master's students and found that gestalt-oriented sandtray "was helpful in increasing supervisee's self-awareness regarding their counselor identity, exploration of new perspectives, and facilitation of acceptance of their struggles and feelings of empowerment" (p. 121).

I have been supervising graduate students and professional counselors for 15 years, and it is one of my favorite professional activities. I feel deep gratitude when I witness a person blossom from being a graduate student, to graduating, to obtaining their licensure as a professional counselor. I have supervised almost every kind of clinician developmentally that exists—master's and doctoral students in practicum, internship, working on pre-licensure hours, and of course, working toward their certification in HST. I have seen sandtray benefit clinicians at every developmental level, whether they are trying to learn how to work with sandtray or using it as an adjunct for personal and professional growth during supervision. Humanistic sandtray can be quite moving for supervisee and supervisor alike in supervision. Because other sandtray therapists have written extensively on the use of sandtray in supervision of counselors and psychotherapists who are not necessarily working toward becoming sandtray therapists (e.g., Homeyer & Lyles, 2022; Homeyer & Sweeney, 2023; Perryman & Anderson, 2011, Perryman et al., 2016; Perryman et al., 2021), my focus in this chapter is something that is discussed infrequently in the sandtray literature: how supervision models and processes apply in supervision of sandtray therapists. My aim is to introduce you to a combined model of supervision that underscores the use of humanistic sandtray supervision in training environments designed to foster development as a humanistic sandtray therapist. I start first, however, with a discussion about the merits of video recording counseling sessions for humanistic sandtray supervision purposes.

The Use of Video Recordings in Supervision

Several models of supervision function best with, and some cannot function at all without, the use of video-recorded counseling sessions (Bernard, 1979, 1997; Kagan & Kagan, 1997; Yontef, 1997). It is simply impossible to know what is going on between a counselor supervisee and their clients without either live supervision or video recording their sessions for review later. Moreover, supervisees are notorious for under-representing or overrepresenting their counseling skills to their supervisors (Bernard & Goodyear, 2019). I have had supervisees report verbally to me what a trainwreck their session was and how they were the worst counselor in the world with a client and, upon my observation of their session, I found myself in total disagreement. It makes pretty good sense that the reason supervisees are under supervision is because they have a limited ability to self-evaluate their counseling approach. One of the primary goals of supervision is to ensure that, by the end of the training period, supervisees can self-supervise because they know what comprises effective counseling.

Therefore, I highly recommend that humanistic sandtray supervisors require their supervisees to video record their counseling sessions. For HST, recording the entire session—from introduction of the sandtray prompt, to the client's selection of miniatures and scene creation process, to the processing phase—allows the supervisor to observe the supervisee's demonstration of appropriate HST skills and assists the supervisee in forming an accurate conceptualization of the client. In addition, as I discuss later in this chapter, there are specific methods of supervision that are integrated into HST that demand the reviewing of the supervisee's video-recorded sessions. If you are an HST supervisor, then your supervisees will need to obtain written permission from their clients in order to video record for supervision purposes. I have included a sample template for such a consent in Appendix C.

Models of Supervision

Bernard and Goodyear (2019) argued that effective supervisors use a three-pronged approach to supervision by synthesizing elements of supervisee development, supervision process, and the supervisor's theory of psychotherapy. Indeed, the HST approach to supervision is anchored in a combined approach with three drivers of supervision: Rønnestad and Skovholt's (2003) lifespan developmental model, Bernard's (1979, 1997) discrimination model, and humanistic-gestalt oriented supervision (Kagan & Kagan, 1997; Yontef, 1997). Each of these models provides direction for supervisors who use humanistic sandtray during supervision and those who supervise humanistic sandtray therapist trainees. The lifespan developmental model (Rønnestad & Skovholt, 2003) acts to normalize supervisees' experiences in various phases of their career, from layperson to experienced therapist. The discrimination model (Bernard, 1979, 1997) provides supervisors with a roadmap for the process of supervision. Humanistic-gestalt oriented supervision concepts (Kagan & Kagan, 1997; Yontef, 1997) bring theoretical elements into the supervisory relationship whereby issues such as parallel process and microawareness are living dynamics between supervisor and supervisee. In this section, I will review each of these models and their application to HST supervision.

Lifespan Developmental Model

Rønnestad and Skovholt's (2003) lifespan developmental model is based on their research with 100 psychotherapists who represented different points along the professional development spectrum, from people who were helpers but had no professional training, to students in their first semester of a mental health therapy training program, to experienced therapists with decades of experience. They discovered that therapists go through six phases over their careers: lay helper, beginning student, advanced student, novice professional, experienced professional, and senior professional.

During the lay helper phase, people engage in non-professionally oriented helper roles such as peers, parents, and work colleagues (Rønnestad & Skovholt, 2003). Their central method of helping is by providing emotional support and advice giving, often projecting their own perceptions and points of view onto the advice they give while also demonstrating significant bias in defense of the person they are helping. Their emotional support often lacks boundaries and they lean into sympathy rather than empathy.

In the beginning student phase, people experience nervous excitement over what is to come in their mental health therapist training (Rønnestad & Skovholt, 2003). They learn a massive amount of information in a relatively short time and sometimes have trouble keeping up with it all. They begin to question long-held assumptions and their self-concept issues become exposed to themselves and their professors. However, as they begin to see their first clients in practicum, they grow most successfully with professors who give them straightforward and constructive feedback while providing positive support. Beginning students take ego hits when they receive negative feedback from clients, just like practitioners who have been seeing clients for years! To help them along the way, students often seek mentors and clinical role models who can provide a vision for the therapist that they want to become. Therefore, it is essential that supervision be a growth-oriented experience consisting of an even mix of support and challenge. Supervision during this phase will set the tone for the rest of the student's career as a clinician.

The third phase is the advanced student phase (Rønnestad & Skovholt, 2003). Advanced students are well into their clinical internships. They continue to feel high anxiety and expect themselves to be better therapists than they are or even could be at this point in their development. As a result, they can be quite sensitive to supervisory feedback. Therefore, as a supervisor, I have found that my level of support with interns needs to match their propensity to assign "shoulds" to operate as perfect clinicians who can solve client issues in three sessions or fewer. One of the more vulnerable aspects of advanced students is that they can sometimes become uncertain about their professional futures because they have strong desires to meet clinical standards of their graduate programs.

Phase four is the novice professional phase (Rønnestad & Skovholt, 2003). During the initial few years after graduating from their graduate mental health degree programs, they seek to "*confirm* the validity of training … [feel] *disillusionment* with professional training and self … [and experience] a more intense *exploration* into self and the professional environment" (p. 17; italics theirs). Although for the first couple of years after graduation novice professionals are under licensure supervision, they still experience a sense of professional freedom. They are no longer under the multiple layers of supervision and close watch that they were during graduate school, and this context leads many to feel excited about their ability to function more independently than ever and scared because they are also more responsible for their own professional trajectory as well as clinical decision-making than ever before. It is the classic existential struggle of freedom versus responsibility. I have noticed that novice professionals under my supervision benefit greatly from validation of their current skillset and opportunities to lean more deeply into engaging in their therapeutic relationships so that they can experience the significance of relational depth to client change.

Phase five is the experienced professional phase (Rønnestad & Skovholt, 2003). Experienced professionals have been practicing therapists for several years. Rønnestad and Skovholt noted that a "central developmental task for most experienced professionals is to create a counseling/therapy role which is highly congruent with the individuals' self-perceptions…and which makes it possible for the practitioner to apply [their] professional competence in an authentic way" (p. 20). Therefore, a major theme during this phase is reflection on how personal experiences influence how individuals operate in their clinical work. For example, I went through a divorce when I was early in the experienced professional phase. It created immediate chaos for me personally, but in the longer term made me a better therapist for clients who are going through relational difficulties and certainly for my work with couples. In addition, experienced professionals demonstrate far more flexibility than during earlier developmental periods. They have integrated who they are into their roles as counselors. They are more boundaried, having learned through experience that leaving their experiences of clients in their consultation rooms at the end of a long workday is optimal for their personal mental health.

Finally, the senior professional phase represents clinicians who are heading toward the sunset of their careers (Rønnestad & Skovholt, 2003). These are clinicians who have practiced for 20 years or more and believe that they have "seen it all." They are experienced with loss, particularly death-related loss, as their professional mentors and perhaps some important colleagues are not as influential as they once were. Common polarities for practitioners in this developmental phase are apathy–inspiration and competence–modesty. Generally, they have intact self-concepts that contribute to a sense of great fulfillment in their role as therapists.

Humanistic Sandtray Supervision and the Lifespan Developmental Model

When practitioners who are working toward their Certified Humanistic Sandtray Therapist (CHST) credential offered by the Humanistic Sandtray Therapy Institute enter the supervision phase of their HST learning process, their developmental level as a therapist impacts their developmental level as a humanistic sandtray therapist. I have supervised individuals working on their CHST credential who are master's students in their clinical internship rotations as well as therapists who have been practicing for ten or more years. Therefore, the supervision process is tailored to the individual's professional development generally as well as their development as a humanistic sandtray therapist. Ultimately, when I am supervising a therapist in their humanistic sandtray work, I adapt my supervisory approach to their lowest developmental level. For example, one of my CHST supervisees had been a practicing counselor for several years and was a phase five experienced professional in terms of his overall therapist development. However, when it came to sandtray, I considered him a phase three advanced student because he had no professional experience using sandtray before he attended my Level I and Level II trainings (see Chapter 12). Therefore, he was brand new to using HST with clients when I began supervising him and had all the typical trappings of an inexperienced sandtray therapist—for example, he expected himself to be better than he was at HST, and because he was an experienced therapist generally, this made the process more complicated and frustrating for him. Therefore, my HST supervisory approach with him mirrored his lowest developmental level, that of an advanced student. The overall message I want to communicate to you is that, when HST supervisors are working with therapists who are learning sandtray, normalizing their developmental needs based on their HST learning process helps them tremendously. Table 13.1 adapts the lifespan developmental model (Rønnestad & Skovholt, 2003) to humanistic sandtray supervision, giving examples of the kinds of dynamics HST supervisors may observe in their supervisees in developmental phases two to five. I have changed the labels of each phase to reflect HST supervisees.

Table 13.1 Supervisory needs of HST supervisees based on the lifespan developmental model (Rønnestad & Skovholt, 2003)

Developmental Phase	HST Training Status	Supervisee Needs in HST
Beginning HST Trainee (R&S Phase 2)	Trainees in HST Levels I and II	Didactic teaching of HST Opportunities to process changes in self-concept (recommend using sandtray). Normalization, support, and encouragement that HST is complex and challenging to learn.
Advanced HST Trainee (R&S Phase 3)	Trainees in individual supervision working on CHST credential	Opportunities to process their anxiety and high self-expectations (recommend using sandtray). Exploration of shoulds. Progress review, noting areas in which supervisee is successfully demonstrating HST.
Novice CHST (R&S Phase 4)	Clinicians who have attained CHST	Consultation to explore advanced methods of applying HST to other formats and populations (groups, couples and families, specialized populations). Exploration of professional self-identity through sandtray.
Experienced CHST (R&S Phase 5)	Clinicians who have been CHSTs for 5 or more years	Opportunities to reflect on and integrate personal experiences into clinical work (recommend using sandtray).

Note: R&S = Rønnestad & Skovholt.

Discrimination Model

The discrimination model (DM; Bernard, 1979, 1997) is commonly used in counselor supervision. Bernard asserted that supervisees benefit from a supervision process in which the roles of the supervisor were clear, and supervisors benefit because they have a roadmap of how to support clinical skill development. When applying the DM, supervisors focus on observing supervisees' intervention, conceptualization, and personalization skills, and facilitate exploration, encouragement, and evaluation. There are three roles that a supervisor assumes at various points in supervision: teacher, counselor, and consultant. As a teacher, supervisors provide direct feedback regarding primarily supervisees' intervention and process skills. They may also introduce their supervisees to knowledge about theory-specific applications. I even consider helping clinicians learn how to write good progress notes as an important part of my teacher role in supervision. When they are in the counselor role, supervisors focus on intrapersonal and interpersonal issues or trends that they observe with their supervisees. These trends may be helping or hindering the counseling process with clients. Armstrong (2008) noted that supervision can be therapeutic, but supervisors are not therapists to their supervisees. The third role of a supervisor is that of consultant. As a supervisee matures professionally, they will require less direct teaching. Therefore, the consultant role emerges over time and experience. The consultant role looks somewhat like peer supervision, in which the supervisor's job is to ask good questions and provoke thought, conceptualization, and discussion with their supervisee.

Humanistic Sandtray Supervision and the Discrimination Model

Carnes-Holt, Meany-Walen, and Felton (2014) discussed their use of sandtray and its application to the DM. They believed that sandtray could be used across each of the supervisor roles of teacher, counselor, and consultant, based upon the supervisee's needs. In the teacher role, Carnes-Holt et al. suggested that supervisors would be teaching and modeling how to use sandtray with clients. In the counselor role, supervisors could use sandtray so that supervisees could process conflicted feelings or countertransference about a client. Finally, in the consultant role, supervisors might provide a prompt for supervisees to identify how they might approach a complex client issue. Carnes-Holt et al. provided a straightforward method to integrate sandtray under the DM, and it aligns well with my approach to HST supervision. Table 13.2 provides example prompts that I have used in the past to assist HST supervisees given each DM role. Of course, there are many other prompts that you can use with your HST and non-HST supervisees based on the DM role that you believe most meets your supervisee's developmental needs.

Table 13.2 Example HST prompts based on discrimination model role

Role	Prompt
Teacher	Create a scene that represents the areas of the humanistic sandtray process about which you feel confused.
	Create a sandtray scene that captures your perception of the therapeutic relationship in humanistic sandtray therapy.
Counselor	Create a sandtray scene that captures how you view yourself as a counselor. Be brutally honest.
	Create a scene that depicts your strengths and how they show up as a counselor.
	Create a sandtray scene that represents your areas of growth and how they show up in your work with clients.
Consultant	Create a world in which you are applying the intervention that would resolve your client's most pressing clinical issues.
	Create a scene that symbolizes the essential elements of the issues with which your client is currently struggling.

Humanistic-Gestalt Elements of Supervision

There are two major psychotherapy theory-based models of supervision that HST supervisors integrate. In this section, I will discuss gestalt supervision (Yontef, 1997) and a humanistic approach to supervision called interpersonal process recall (Kagan & Kagan, 1997). Then, I will discuss how these models apply to HST supervision.

Gestalt Supervision

In some ways, gestalt supervision mirrors the gestalt psychotherapy process (Yontef, 1997). This is not to say that gestalt supervision is undercover psychotherapy; on the contrary, when supervisors have an important administrative role such as employer or professor and are responsible for evaluation of a supervisee's career or performance in a graduate program, Yontef noted that the experiential nature of supervision would be significantly limited so as not to violate ethical codes. However, processes such as contact, contact boundaries, the paradoxical theory of change, and field theory all operate within the supervisory relationship because these are human, organismic dynamics and cannot be separated from psychotherapy supervision.

The overall goal of supervision is to contribute to the growth of the supervisee and their clients (Yontef, 1997). Because increased awareness takes place based on the quality of contact, supervisors attempt to be in contact with self and supervisee and assist the supervisee in making good contact with their clients. In terms of awareness, of significant focus in gestalt supervision is working with supervisees with their own microawareness as it applies to their clinical work and therapeutic relationships. Similarly, gestalt supervisors view supervisee change as paradoxical; therefore, of particular focus is encouraging supervisees to identify who they are instead of who they are not, both in the supervisory relationship and, more meaningfully, in their therapeutic relationships.

Speaking of change, Yontef (1997) discussed resistance, or interference, as a natural part of supervision. He identified three examples of interference. The first consists of "unrealistic expectations by the supervisor, supervisee, or agency" (p. 162); this form of interference shows up when the supervisor provides, or the supervisee expects, easy answers to complicated clinical matters. Unrealistic expectations can also drive supervisees to refer or terminate challenging clients, and supervisors may not put in efforts to help supervisees improve their work with higher-need clients. A second example of interference appears when supervisors have a "narcissistic need" (p. 162) to be worshipped by their supervisees without recognizing or admitting to this need. When supervisors are wrapped up in their own ego, they tend to place supervisee and client needs lower, and this dysfunctional rearrangement of whose needs take precedence can mean an imbalance of power whereby both the supervisee's training needs suffer and potentially the client's therapeutic needs are ignored. A third example of interference happens when either supervisor or supervisee, or both, simply do not want to engage in supervision. This interference is particularly troublesome when supervisors or supervisees are meeting for supervision because they are required to or because of training or employer requirements.

Field theory provides that supervision takes place in context. Therefore, Yontef (1997) identified three major contexts of gestalt supervision: administrative, educative, and consultative. During administrative supervision, gestalt supervisors help supervisees with fulfilling the requirements of the field in which they provide therapy, such as an agency setting, a university counseling center, or a private practice. Supervisors provide direction for supervisees to follow legal and ethical standards, workplace policies, and licensure or training requirements. Supervisors expose supervisees to the nature of hierarchies, systems, and social and political issues as applicable to their clinical setting. In addition, supervisors remain open to hearing and providing support to supervisees' experiences regarding the impact of the many policies, codes, laws, hierarchies, and systems on supervisees. The educative function of gestalt supervision is similar to the teacher role in the DM with an obvious focus on teaching gestalt methods. Finally, the consultative function provides a framework for supervisors to attend to the specific growth-oriented needs of their supervisees. During consultation, there are three major foci: effective psychotherapy methods (both general and theory-specific); client conceptualization and therapeutic needs; and supervisee self-understanding and awareness.

Interpersonal Process Recall: A Humanistic Model

The interpersonal process recall (IPR; Kagan & Kagan, 1997) model is a humanistic-phenomenological structured supervision approach in which supervisors and supervisees collaborate to discover and explore the supervisee's hidden emotions that arise when working with clients. IPR is implemented in the here and now in the safe environment of clinical supervision. The basic process of IPR goes like this:

1. The supervisor and the supervisee watch a video-recorded counseling session together.
2. Either the supervisor or the supervisee pauses the video. The supervisor prompts the supervisee to express what the supervisee was feeling or thinking at the exact time of the session.
3. The supervisor invites the supervisee to re-experience that moment of their counseling session.

Of course, the process itself is a little more complex than what I have described. The supervisor should act as a co-explorer. They should be in a non-evaluative and non-judgmental mode during IPR. During IPR, I tend to invite my supervisee into sensory-emotional awareness. For example, I might say, "What are you feeling at this moment as the client is welling up with tears?" IPR can have an important part to play in increasing awareness of supervisees' emotional experiencing while they are with clients, and they might discover some unfinished business along the way. It can be used in an individual, triadic, or group setting. In triadic and group settings, I often open it up to others in the supervision group to explore their reactions to what they are observing in a peer's video-recorded counseling session.

Humanistic Sandtray Supervision and Humanistic-Gestalt Elements

HST supervisors are theoretically undergirded by humanistic-gestalt elements of supervision. As an HST supervisor, I open myself to contact with my supervisees and my sense of self. When I am working with supervisees, I am operating in three overlapping fields: administrative; educative; and consultative. When I operate within the administrative field of supervision, I help my supervisees navigate requirements of licensing if applicable and the HST certification process, as well as ethical or legal dilemmas that may arise during their work with clients. Often these issues can be captured through discussion; however, it can be a real advantage when my clients place their world of administrative hurdles in the tray. For example, HST supervisors could prompt a supervisee who is struggling with an ethical dilemma to create a sandtray scene that captures the essence of their impasse. It can assist the decision-making process and nudge them toward action.

Within the educative field, I teach HST trainees the requisite therapeutic principles, skills, and methodology of HST. Principally, I function in this context during the HST Level I and Level II trainings, as this is when I am in full teaching mode and exposing trainees to concepts that may be new to them. Certainly, the educative field involves a fundamentally didactic process.

Finally, the consultative field provides an opportunity for me to work with supervisees to improve their HST-specific skills, methods, and process approach. Commonly, my supervisees bring in a video-recorded sandtray session with a client and I offer corrective feedback to their HST approach. My feedback might center on practical issues such as their sandtray collection or the prompt they provided their client. More commonly, I focus on their HST process skills. Like the administrative component, it is typical for me to ask my supervisee to create a sandtray scene in order to model the HST approach in real time. Also, supervisees may create sandtray scenes that represent how they theoretically conceptualize their clients. Other times, supervisees create sandtrays to explore self and encourage microawareness of their intrapersonal reactions to clients.

Kagan and Kagan's (1997) IPR is an excellent fit for opening a space for supervisees to become familiar with microawareness. Remember that Yontef (1993) defined microawareness as generating awareness of awareness. Microawareness is an essential process to humanistic sandtray therapist supervisees because it allows them to discover their emotional reactions to self as well as their clients. Because IPR is designed to provide a structure for here-and-now exploration of these dynamics, I recommend that HST supervisors use a modified version of it. Here is how I tend to facilitate an HST supervision session using IPR:

1. My supervisee and I watch a video-recorded HST session that my supervisee recently had with a client.
2. One of us pauses the video when one of us notices a potential emotional response or reaction from the supervisee during their counseling session. Regardless of who initiates pausing the video, I provide a sandtray

prompt that seems related to what is happening in the moment of the video. An example might be, "It seems like something is coming up for you in this moment in your session. Create a sandtray scene that depicts what is coming up for you there."

3. The supervisee and I enter into a processing phase of the sandtray, which invites the supervisee to experience and explore what was happening during the session in the here and now.

In my experience, IPR is a natural fit for the gestalt elements that I have adapted to HST supervision.

A Combined Model of Humanistic Sandtray Supervision

HST supervisors use a combined model of supervision as suggested by Bernard and Goodyear (2019). From a practical point of view, here is how each model contributes to supervision of humanistic sandtray therapists:

1. Throughout the process of supervision, the HST supervisor creates and maintains an effective supervisory alliance and relationship by co-creating contact.

2. An HST supervisor observes cues from their supervisee's overall intra and interpersonal functioning, patterns, needs, and behaviors during supervision and counseling, noting similarities and differences that take place during traditional talk therapy and sandtray therapy.

3. The HST supervisor's observations form the basis of the conceptualization of the supervisee's developmental phase according to Rønnestad and Skovholt's (2003) lifespan developmental model. The supervisee's developmental phase may differ between their overall development as a therapist and development specific to HST.

4. The HST supervisor creates a supervision plan and responds to the supervisee based on the supervisee's idiosyncratic way of living out their developmental phase and needs with respect to their emergence as a humanistic sandtray therapist and the requisite attitudes, skills, and dynamics. Each supervision session, the HST supervisor intentionally responds in a supervisory role, that of teacher, counselor, or consultant, based in the DM (Bernard, 1979, 1997) and with respect to the existing context of administrative, educative, and consultative (Yontef, 1997), providing the supervisee opportunities to engage in IPR when appropriate. The supervisor's role must be congruent with the supervisee's needs-in-context as a humanistic sandtray therapist in training.

With these four qualities of HST supervision in mind, I review a supervision session I had with one of my HST supervisees in Case Study 13.1.

Case Study 13.1: Hudson

Hudson is one of my supervisees working toward his licensed professional counselor status as well as his CHST. He was one of my graduate students, and I trained him in HST. I have supervised him individually for over two years, first during his graduate internship at a middle school at which he used HST as the therapeutic medium, and now he is employed at a local mental health agency providing in-home counseling with clients with disabilities.

During one recent supervision session, Hudson asked me, "How do I come up with good sandtray prompts for clients that go beyond the broad HST ones?" I told him that one of the best ways for me to answer his question was to demonstrate it with him. I suggested that he discuss something he had been struggling with lately pursuant to therapeutic relationships with clients and that would help me come up with a sandtray prompt that would be responsive to his need. He stated that he had been thinking about his role and impact on his clients and seemed tenuous about both. I asked him to talk about this issue in terms of his current clients. Two clients came up for him. One was a female client with a stepmom whom she despised. Another was a male client who often seemed stuck in decision-making.

I presented an idea for a sandtray prompt. I summarized his question and asked him to create a scene in the sandtray that captured how he views his own responsibility in the therapeutic relationship and for client change. He created his sandtray scene and, before we discussed his scene, I explained to him that sandtray prompts can be very broad at first, but as the therapist gets to know the client and their context, effective prompts can be based off of the content of the client's concern during any one session.

Then, I asked Hudson to describe his scene. Hudson told me that while creating his scene, he was thinking to himself, "What am I bringing to this therapeutic relationship?" He chose a generic-looking figure to represent himself, surrounded by books and two trees. He said that he saw his role as, "I'm just here. Clients are living the journey of their life. They just happened to run into me. I'm trying to use these few little tools I've picked up through training and school to work with clients." He placed two figures in his scene representing specific clients—one was Pinocchio and the other was a blue-haired fairy. Hudson made a giant X in the sand representing pathways crossing, and the figure representing him was in the middle. The client figures were facing him.

I responded, "Sounds like you have a fear of being successful." Hudson responded affirmatively and talked in detail about being arrogant as an adolescent, which led to a series of bad relationships. He discovered that arrogance got him "nothing in life." He told me that he was afraid of going back to that part of him in which he would convince himself that he knew how people should live their lives. He was afraid of bringing those characteristics into his therapeutic relationships.

I offered a potential polarity within Hudson. He wanted to be an important part of his clients' lives, and he was afraid that he would do so in an ego-driven way. I encouraged him to acknowledge the narcissistic side of him. In addition, I said, "That is clearly not who you are; that is a façade that you created. You were acting."

In response, Hudson expressed wanting to change the figure. He changed it to a figure that represented a hero. As we further processed his revised sandtray scene, Hudson described his internal experiencing as a metaphor, changing from a young Aragorn from *The Lord of the Rings*, who felt an unworthy need to reconcile sins from the past to a matured Aragorn who accepted that he could do more than be an anonymous hero. He told me that he felt a sense that it was okay to be more than just a milquetoast therapist. He suggested that it was okay to recognize that he was having an impact on people's lives. He stated that he felt a sense of acceptance for what he wanted his role in his clients' lives to be—an active and compassionate therapist who walked alongside his clients and helped to expose them to new ways of experiencing and making choices.

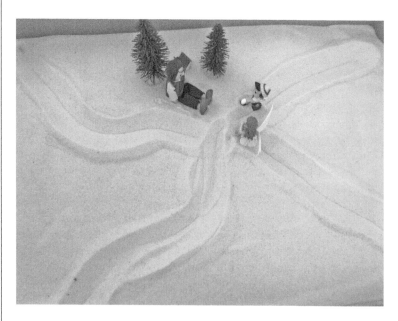

Figure 13.1 Sandtray created during humanistic sandtray supervision.

Group Humanistic Sandtray Supervision

Thus far, I have discussed individual HST supervision. However, group supervision is an especially profitable environment in which to use sandtray (Homeyer & Sweeney, 2023). Bernard and Goodyear (2019) noted a number of advantages to group supervision; these benefits apply to HST supervision groups, too. It can be cost effective for HST supervisees not just financially but also in terms of time. In addition, groups provide HST supervisees with opportunities for vicarious learning—supervisees learn from feedback that other group members receive from the HST supervisor and each other. Relatedly, groups offer HST supervisees exposure to clients and client issues that they may not experience in their own clinical setting, and they can discuss different ways of approaching sandtray therapy. An obvious benefit is that supervisees get feedback from other group members, which exposes them to a tremendously valuable diversity of clinical experience and settings. Moreover, an HST supervision group allows the supervisor to see additional aspects of a supervisee's intra and interpersonal processes due to the nature of group dynamics. Also, group supervisees can observe HST supervision skills when other supervisees are the focus of feedback. Group supervision can normalize supervisees' frustrations and struggles with developing into a good humanistic sandtray therapist, too. Finally, some elements of HST group supervision can mirror that of clinical HST groups, exposing supervisees to methods of using HST in a group format. Effective group HST supervisors integrate what I have presented in this chapter in terms of a combined model of HST supervision with characteristics and dynamics of HST groups that I discussed in Chapter 9.

Conclusion

Supervision is a critical part of the development of counselors who are training to become humanistic sandtray therapists. HST supervision is founded upon a combined model influenced by the lifespan developmental model (Rønnestad & Skovholt, 2003), the discrimination model (Bernard, 1979, 1997), gestalt supervision (Yontef, 1997), and IPR (Kagan & Kagan, 1997). A key requirement of HST supervision is the video recording of supervisees' counseling sessions. Although HST supervision takes place primarily with individual supervisees, a group format can be an effective adjunct to individual supervision.

References

Armstrong, S. A. (2008). *Sandtray therapy: A humanistic approach*. Ludic Press.

Bernard, J. M. (1979). Supervisor training: A discrimination model. *Counselor Education and Supervision*, 19, 60–68. https://doi.org/10.1002/j.1556-6978.1979.tb00906.x

Bernard, J. M. (1997). The discrimination model. In C. E. Watkins, Jr. (Ed.), *Handbook of psychotherapy supervision* (pp. 310–327). Wiley.

Bernard, J. M., & Goodyear, R. K. (2019). *Fundamentals of clinical supervision* (6th ed.). Pearson.

Carnes-Holt, K., Meany-Walen, K., & Felton, A. (2014). Utilizing sandtray within the discrimination model of counselor supervision. *Journal of Creativity in Mental Health, 9*(4), 497–510. https://doi.org/10.1080/15401383.2014.909298

Casado-Kehoe, M., & Ybañez-Llorente, K. (2018). Clinical supervision. In S. Degges-White & N. L. Davis (Eds.), *Integrating the expressive arts into counseling practice: Theory-based interventions* (2nd ed., pp. 259–267). Springer.

Homeyer, L. E., & Lyles, M. N. (2022). *Advanced sandtray therapy: Digging deeper into clinical practice.* Routledge. https://doi.org/10.4324/9781003095491

Homeyer, L. E., & Sweeney, D. S. (2023). *Sandtray therapy: A practical manual* (4th ed.). Routledge. https://doi.org/10.4324/9781003221418

Kagan, H. K., & Kagan, N. I. (1997). Interpersonal process recall: Influencing human interaction. In C. E. Watkins, Jr. (Ed.), *Handbook of psychotherapy supervision* (pp. 296–309). Wiley.

Loganbill, C., Hardy, E., & Delworth, U. (1982). Supervision: A conceptual model. *Counseling Psychologist, 10*(1), 3–42. https://doi.org/10.1177/001100008 2101002

Newsome, D. W., Henderson, D. A., & Veach, L. J. (2011). Using expressive arts in group supervision to enhance awareness and foster cohesion. *The Journal of Humanistic Counseling, 44*(2), 145–157. https://doi.org/10.1002/j.2164-490X.2005.tb00027.x

Perryman, K., & Anderson, A. (2011). Using sandtray in supervision. In S. Degges-White & N. Davis, (Eds.), *Integrating the expressive arts into counseling practice: Theory-based intervention* (pp. 241–248). Springer.

Perryman, K. L., Moss, R. C., & Anderson, L. (2016). Sandtray supervision: An integrated model for play therapy supervision. *International Journal of Play Therapy, 25*(4), 186–196. https://doi.org/10.1037/pla0040288

Perryman, K. L., Houin, C. B., Leslie, T. N., & Finley, S. K. (2021). Using sandtray as a creative supervision tool. *Journal of Creativity in Mental Health, 16*(1), 109–124. https://doi.org/10.1080/15401383.2020.1754988

Rønnestad, M. H., & Skovholt, T. M. (2003). The journey of the counselor and therapist: Research findings and perspectives on professional development. *Journal of Career Development, 30*(1), 5–44. https://doi.org/10.1023/A:1025173508081

Stoltenberg, C. D., McNeill, B. W., & Delworth, U. (1998). *IDM: An integrated developmental model for supervising counselors and therapists.* Jossey-Bass.

Yontef, G. (1993). *Awareness, dialogue & process.* The Gestalt Press.

Yontef, G. (1997). Supervision from a gestalt therapy perspective. In C. E. Watkins, Jr. (Ed.), *Handbook of psychotherapy supervision* (pp. 147–163). Wiley.

Chapter 14

Sandtray Therapy Research

Research is one of the most prominent ways that psychotherapists can support with veracity that what they do works for the populations they serve. In the modern environment of lifting the once mysterious veil of what happens in therapy and how it works for clients and the public to observe, therapists have an ethical responsibility to use approaches that are part of the growing compendium of evidence-based practices (American Counseling Association, 2014). The American Psychological Association (APA) Presidential Task Force on Evidence-Based Practice (2006) defined evidence-based practice as "the integration of the best available research with clinical expertise in the context of patient characteristics, culture, and preferences" (p. 273). For the purposes of this chapter, I will focus on the first pillar, that of research. By "best available research," they meant that clinical practices should have an established record of published research consisting of many different methodologies and designs. The APA endorses a wide range of research types, including case studies, single-case designs, qualitative research, process studies, meta-analyses, and randomized controlled trials (RCTs). In addition, research should take place in a variety of settings, including laboratory and field/naturalistic settings.

In my opinion, sand therapists, regardless of theoretical background, have a professional obligation to ensure that our practices are evidence-based. There is a growing number of RCTs that demonstrate strong evidence for the therapeutic impact of sandplay therapy on a wide array of clients and presenting issues (Roesler, 2019). In addition, several meta-analyses have demonstrated the effectiveness of sandplay therapy (Lee & Jang, 2015; Koh & Ha, 2022; Wiersma et al., 2022). Unfortunately, sandtray therapy is not considered an evidence-based practice and has a long way to go to establish it as such. In this chapter, I will summarize the existing quantitative evidence supporting sandtray therapy broadly and provide a roadmap for researchers who have interest in generating evidentiary support for HST.

DOI: 10.4324/9781032664996-18

A Summary of Sandtray Therapy Research Studies

A colleague of mine and I published a meta-analysis on sand therapies and included both sandplay and sandtray studies (Holliman & Foster, 2023). To be included in our meta-analysis, we established the following criteria: "(1) intervention study using sand therapy; (2) quantitative data collected; (3) sufficient statistics to calculate effect size; and (4) written in English" (p. 208). We investigated several research questions. First, we wanted to know the overall efficacy of sand therapy interventions. Second, we wanted to know if age impacted efficacy of sand therapy interventions. Third, we wanted to know if the format of sand therapy interventions—specifically, individual or group—impacted their efficacy. Finally, we wanted to know the efficacy of sand therapy on anxiety, depression, anger, self-esteem, and parent–child relationships. We discovered that, generally, sand therapy interventions were efficacious across a broad range of client presenting issues. In addition, we found that sand therapies were effective interventions for depression, anxiety, and parent–child relationship issues. We found no differences in the efficacy of sand therapies based on age or format. Our results were similar to prior sandplay meta-analyses (e.g., Lee & Jang, 2015; Koh & Ha, 2022; Wiersma et al., 2022).

A Call to the Field of Sandtray Therapy

Here is the part that stood out to me when my colleague and I performed our analysis. Out of a total of 36 sand therapy studies, we located only four sandtray treatment outcome studies that met our criteria—the remaining 32 were sandplay (Holliman & Foster, 2023). You read that right: *four* (see Table 14.1 for a summary of these studies). That is not very many, particularly considering how long sandtray has been around. Frankly, there is a scant amount of treatment outcome research supporting the effectiveness of sandtray therapy. If you perform a Google Scholar search, you will find plenty of case examples of sandtray. However, the field of sandtray therapy is nowhere close to consideration as an evidence-based practice according to the APA's (2006) guidelines.

Table 14.1 Summary of sandtray therapy treatment outcome studies

Study	N	Population	Outcome Assessed	Sandtray Theory/ Approach	Intervention Format
Flahive & Ray, 2007	56	Children with behavioral issues	Problematic behaviors, externalizing problems, internalizing problems	Unidentified	Group

Table 14.1 (Continued)

Study	N	Population	Outcome Assessed	Sandtray Theory/ Approach	Intervention Format
Nelson-Ray, 2007	77	At-risk adolescents	Academic achievement, school satisfaction, problematic behaviors, school attendance rates	The World Technique	Group
Plotkin, 2011	32	Children who were experiencing parental divorce	Internalizing problems, externalizing problems	Child-centered	Individual
Shen & Armstrong, 2008	37	Adolescent girls with low self-esteem	Self-esteem	Humanistic	Group

My purpose in using such direct language in identifying this paucity of methodologically sound treatment outcome research investigating sandtray interventions is to make a resounding call to the sandtray therapy field and its associated researchers to generate methodologically strong efficacy and effectiveness investigations. In particular, I am interested in establishing HST as an evidence-based practice. Therefore, to assist my fellow researchers with designing treatment outcome studies on HST, I developed the *Humanistic Sandtray Therapy Treatment Manual* (Foster, 2024), which I have included as Appendix D in this book. You may also access this treatment manual on the Humanistic Sandtray Therapy Institute's website at https://humanisticsandtray.com. If you are interested in designing such research studies on HST, you have open permission to use my treatment manual to assist you.

Conclusion

If I get the opportunity to write further revised editions of this book, I hope that this chapter will be longer. I hope that investigators begin to generate more rigorous, and a greater quantity of, research studies on sandtray therapy interventions, including but not limited to HST. Like many of you, I have witnessed the power of sandtray therapy with my clients and my supervisees' clients. I know that sandtray helps heal wounded clients. To establish HST as an evidence-based practice, a more formal exploration of its effect and efficacy is needed.

References

American Counseling Association. (2014). *Code of ethics*. Author. https://www.cou nseling.org/resources/aca-code-of-ethics.pdf

APA Presidential Task Force on Evidence-Based Practice. (2006). Evidence-based practice in psychology. *American Psychologist, 61*(4), 271–285. https://doi.org/ 10.1037/0003-066X.61.4.271

Flahive, M. H. W., & Ray, D. (2007). Effect of group sandtray therapy with preadolescents. *The Journal for Specialists in Group Work, 32*(4), 362–382. https://doi. org/10.1080/01933920701476706

Foster, R. D. (2024). *Humanistic sandtray therapy treatment manual*. Humanistic Sandtray Therapy Institute.

Holliman, R., & Foster, R. D. (2023). The way we play in the sand: A meta-analytic investigation of sand therapy, its formats, and presenting problems. *Journal of Child and Adolescent Counseling, 9*(2), 205–221. https://doi.org/10.1080/ 23727810.2023.2232142

Koh, H., & Ha, J. (2022). A meta-analysis on the effectiveness of sand play therapy in adults. *Journal of Symbols & Sandplay Therapy, 13*(2), 137–156. https://doi. org/10.12964/jsst.22009

Lee, J.-S., & Jang, D.-H. (2015). The effectiveness of sand play treatment metaanalysis. *Korean Journal of Child Psychological Therapy, 10*(1), 1–26.

Nelson-Ray, P. (2007). *Using sand tray with at-risk students to impact school success* [Unpublished doctoral dissertation]. Texas Tech University.

Plotkin, L. (2011). Children's adjustment following parental divorce: How effective is sandtray therapy? [Unpublished doctoral dissertation]. Capella University.

Roesler, C. (2019). Sandplay therapy: An overview of theory, applications and evidence base. *The Arts in Psychotherapy, 64*, 84–94. https://doi.org/10.1016/ j.aip.2019.04.001

Shen, Y. P., & Armstrong, S. A. (2008). Impact of group sandtray therapy on the self-esteem of young adolescent girls. *The Journal for Specialists in Group Work, 33*(2), 118–137. https://doi.org/10.1080/01933920801977397

Wiersma, J. K., Freedle, L. R., McRoberts, R., & Solberg, K. B. (2022). A metaanalysis of sandplay therapy treatment outcomes. *International Journal of Play Therapy, 31*(4), 197–215. https://doi.org/10.1037/pla0000180

Chapter 15

Contemporary Issues and Future Directions

In 2008, Steve Armstrong established the foundation for HST with the publication of *Sandtray Therapy: A Humanistic Approach*. I hope that my expansion of the underlying philosophy, therapeutic conditions, and essentials of the real therapeutic relationship as they pertain to HST continues to broaden the influence of this model on therapists who are looking for a structured, theoretically sound, and flexible method to apply to their sandtray practice. Mostly, I hope that clients who work with humanistic sandtray therapists experience the profound benefits that I have witnessed in my own clinical work. As Yontef (1993) pointed out, theories and models are dynamic and multidimensional, so I know that as a wider community of scholar-practitioners use and evaluate various aspects of HST, more will be discovered about what makes it effective practice. In this chapter, I will share my thoughts about the present and the future of sandtray.

Sand Therapy Competencies

HST shares common elements of all sand therapies. Homeyer and Stone (2023) reported results of their survey of sand therapy professionals and identified a number of content knowledge areas and qualities of sand therapists. A majority of respondents reported that sand therapists should have knowledge of sand therapy theory, human development, psychopathology, anti-discriminatory therapeutic approaches, research, and systemic theories. Hartwig, Homeyer, and Stone (2023) discussed results of a qualitative study in which their goal was to more deeply explore universal competencies for sand therapists regardless of theoretical disposition. Their investigation resulted in a model that included 33 competencies categorized in four major areas: knowledge, skills, attitudes, and professional engagement. HST, as I have presented in this book, is inclusive of all 33 competencies. This overlap bodes well for practitioners who are looking to adopt a model of sandtray therapy that is undergirded by professional competencies based in evidence.

DOI: 10.4324/9781032664996-19

HST Applications and Research

There is more yet to be discovered about applications of HST. I invite you to explore new ways of applying HST to populations, clinical settings, and therapy formats that I did not discuss in this text. In particular, I hope to learn even more about how HST can be adapted to diverse clients, couples, families, and groups. Moreover, although HST is a non-pathologizing approach, mental health diagnoses form a common language for clinicians to understand the ways in which clients' emotional experiencing can influence problematic thinking and behaviors, and some diagnoses have biological etiologies. Therefore, I would like to discover ways in which HST impacts various diagnoses. Relatedly, one of my major goals is to establish HST as an evidence-based practice, which requires dedicated sandtray researchers to carry out methodologically sound scholarly investigations. One avenue is to investigate treatment outcome of HST on focused diagnostic categories. Although I have my own research studies currently in progress, I cannot build this evidence base all by myself!

Ethics of Sandtray Therapy

One last piece that I believe needs to be established in the sandtray therapy community is a code of ethics. Sandplay therapists have explored ethical issues around their method (Loue, 2015), and although many of the ethical issues they discussed likely mirror those of sandtray therapy, there are major differences between the two schools of sand therapy. Having a sandtray therapy code of ethics would help with developing global standards of care for this practice. It would also help instill confidence in practitioners and clients alike that sandtray therapists take ethical issues seriously.

Conclusion

As you and I come to the close of this text, I am in deep reflection about the impact that HST has had on me, personally. Moreover, in my mind's eye I can see the many clients with whom I have facilitated sandtray and their pain, growth, and healing. Having engaged on both sides of the tray, I value my experiences in the sand, and I am aware of a holistic sense of gratitude for the world of the sandtray. Humanistic sandtray therapy is an experience and a process; a collection of moments, dynamics, and defenses; an opportunity for awareness, microawareness, and paradoxical change; and a meaningful space for discovery and exploration.

References

Armstrong, S. A. (2008). *Sandtray therapy: A humanistic approach*. Ludic Press.

Hartwig, E. K., Homeyer, L. E., & Stone, J. (2023). Sand therapy competencies: A qualitative investigation of competencies for sand therapy practitioners. *World Journal for Sand Therapy Practice*, *1*(5), 1–20. https://doi.org/10.58997/wjstp.v1i5.32

Homeyer, L. E., & Stone, J. (2023). Sand therapy standards: Views from the field. *World Journal for Sand Therapy Practice*, *1*(1), 1–11. https://doi.org/10.58997/wjstp.v1i1.4

Loue, S. (Ed.). (2015). *Ethical issues in sandplay therapy practice and research.* Springer.

Yontef, G. (1993). *Awareness, dialogue and process.* The Gestalt Press.

Appendices

Appendix A

Humanistic Sandtray Therapy Progress Note

Therapist: _____ Client: _____ Age: _____

Date of Session: _____ Time: _____ Session #: ___

Diagnosis (ICD-10-CM): _____ CPT Code: _____

Data:

Client Presentation/Appearance: ☐Appropriate ☐Unkempt ☐Poor hygiene ☐Other:___

Affect and Mood: ☐Congruent ☐Incongruent ☐Labile ☐Heightened ☐Depressed

☐Full range ☐Constricted ☐Anxious ☐Dysphoric ☐Apathetic ☐Angry/Irritable

☐Calm ☐Joyful ☐Other: _____

Safety Concerns: ☐Denies SI ☐Denies self-harm ☐Denies HI ☐Other: _____

Sandtray Prompt Used:

Topics Discussed: ☐School ☐Parents ☐Siblings ☐Friends/Peers ☐Romantic relationships
☐Work ☐Others: _____

Interventions Used: ☐Sandtray creation ☐Reflection of feeling/meaning

☐ Centering exercise ☐Here-and-now/immediacy ☐Guided into immediate emotion

☐ Stayed with emotion ☐Went deeper into emotion ☐Accentuated the obvious

☐ Facilitated ownership of experiences/I-language ☐Enactment ☐Body awareness

☐ Worked with metaphor in the sand tray ☐Polarities: Identified, named, and
acknowledged ☐Polarities: Separated and explored ☐Polarities: Facilitated
acceptance of both parts ☐Polarities: Facilitated integration of parts ☐Worked
with resistance

Copyright material from Ryan D. Foster (2025), *Humanistic Sandtray Therapy*, Routledge

Categories of Sandtray Miniatures Used and Significance:

☐ People: _____

☐ Animals: _____

☐ Buildings: _____

☐ Transportation: _____

☐ Vegetation: _____

☐ Fences/gates/signs: _____

☐ Natural items: _____

☐ Fantasy: _____

☐ Spiritual/mystical: _____

☐ Landscaping and other accessories: _____

☐ Household items: _____

☐ Multicultural/diversity-oriented: _____

☐ Other: _____

Copyright material from Ryan D. Foster (2025), *Humanistic Sandtray Therapy*, Routledge

ATTACH DIGITAL PHOTOGRAPH OF SAND TRAY TO PROGRESS NOTE

Assessment:

Disposition of the Therapeutic Relationship:

Polarities Explored:

Summary of Metaphors in the Tray (including any progress in metaphors noted):

Contact Boundary Disturbances Noted:

☐ Retroflection ☐ Introjection ☐ Projection ☐ Deflection

Conceptualization and Progress:

Plan:

Next Scheduled Session

Date and Time: _____

Location: ☐ Virtual ☐ In-Office ☐ Other: _____

Referrals Provided:

Other Information:

Copyright material from Ryan D. Foster (2025), *Humanistic Sandtray Therapy*, Routledge

Appendix B

Informed Consent for Humanistic Sandtray Therapy

Qualifications: I have a Doctor of Philosophy (PhD) in Counseling from the University of North Texas. I am a Licensed Professional Counselor-Supervisor (LPC-S; #63186) in the State of Texas and a Certified Humanistic Sandtray Therapist (CHST). Based on my LPC licensure, I am qualified to provide counseling and psychological assessment services independently in Texas. My formal education and training have prepared me to counsel individual adults, adolescents, children, couples, families, and groups with a variety of concerns.

Experience: I have counseled children, adolescents, adults, couples, families, and groups. I have experience and professional training in using expressive therapies such as play therapy, expressive arts, and dreamwork. I also have advanced training in grief and loss counseling. In addition, I have extensive training and experience in using sandtray therapy.

About Sandtray Therapy: I am a Certified Humanistic Sandtray Therapist (CHST), which means that I have advanced training in an experiential method of psychotherapy called *humanistic sandtray therapy* (HST). In HST, clients create a scene in a sandtray using a collection of miniature figures. The scene is meant to symbolize some part of a client's life, struggles they may be going through, goals that they may have, or experiences that they are going through. If I believe HST might be helpful to you during the course of therapy, then I will invite you to have an open discussion about it.

If you and I agree that HST might be helpful, then my hope is that you will discover parts of yourself of which you were previously unaware and use your increasing self-awareness to experience your whole self—body, mind, and heart. Your experiences and awareness may lead to growth and change; however, any changes, no matter how major or minor, will always be left up to you to choose.

Copyright material from Ryan D. Foster (2025), *Humanistic Sandtray Therapy*, Routledge

Effects of Sandtray Therapy: At any time, you may initiate with me a discussion of possible positive or negative effects of entering or not entering, continuing, or discontinuing humanistic sandtray therapy. I expect you to benefit from sandtray. However, I cannot guarantee any specific results. Humanistic sandtray therapy is a personal exploration that may lead to major changes in your life perspectives and decisions. These changes may affect significant relationships, your job or educational environment, and/or your understanding of yourself. You may feel troubled, usually only temporarily, by some of the things you learn about yourself or some of the changes you make. In addition, sandtray therapy can, at times, result in long lasting effects. For example, one risk of exploring intimate relationships during sandtray therapy is the possibility that the relationship may end. Although the exact nature of changes resulting from humanistic sandtray therapy cannot be predicted, I intend to work with you to achieve the best possible results for you.

Photographs of Your Sandtray: I encourage my clients to take photographs of their own sandtrays so that they may continue to reflect on their experience. I also take a digital photo of your sandtray scene and attach it to my session notes as part of your electronic health records.

Copyright material from Ryan D. Foster (2025), *Humanistic Sandtray Therapy*, Routledge

Appendix C

Permission to Video Record Humanistic Sandtray Therapy Sessions

I _____ consent to the video recording of therapy sessions with
(Client name) Ryan D. Foster, PhD, LPC-S, CHST. I am aware of the presence of the video equipment and permit the use of all or part of the video recording for the purpose of:

_____ My therapist's consultation with a clinical supervisor(s)
(Client initials) and/or training group.

In no way will the refusal to grant consent for this video recording affect my therapeutic care. If at any time during the treatment process, I wish to stop the recording, I may do so and continue treatment. All recordings are considered confidential material and will be treated with professional respect and courtesy according to the Texas LPC Code of Ethics, Texas state laws, and the American Counseling Association Code of Ethics. Recordings will be deleted after review. Video recordings are not part of client files.

_____   _____
Client Signature   Date

_____   _____
Therapist Signature   Date

Copyright material from Ryan D. Foster (2025), *Humanistic Sandtray Therapy*, Routledge

Appendix D

Humanistic Sandtray Therapy Treatment Manual

Theoretical Overview of Humanistic Sandtray Therapy

Sandtray therapy is an umbrella term that captures various theoretical and cross-theoretical approaches (Homeyer & Sweeney, 2023). Humanistic sandtray therapy (HST) is defined as *a dynamic, experiential philosophical approach to sandtray therapy grounded in a synthesis of person-centered and gestalt theories in which the power of the here and now is harnessed to invite clients into increased awareness and paradoxical change*. The goal of HST is to facilitate increased awareness of clients' immediate emotional experiencing and resulting emotional, cognitive, and/or behavioral responses or reactions to self and environment.

Armstrong (2008) described first his humanistic approach as an integration of person-centered and gestalt theories. Foster (2025) expanded this model to further delineate the theoretical mechanisms underlying HST. Person-centered gestaltists value the following tenets:

1. A Maslovian foundation based on the self-actualizing tendency.
2. The value of discovery learning.
3. The essence of the therapeutic process as experiencing.
4. Emphasis on the creation of an authentic and trusting I/Thou relationship.
5. Attention to the genuineness of the therapist as a person.
6. The need for therapists to be with clients while retaining their own separateness.
7. The belief that their approaches, widely applied, would benefit both the individual and society (Herlihy, 1985, p. 21).

In addition, HST aligns with humanistic theories in their understanding of human nature and the capacities with which people are born into the world:

Copyright material from Ryan D. Foster (2025), *Humanistic Sandtray Therapy*, Routledge

1. *Actualizing and self-actualizing tendency:* Innately, people feel propelled toward growth, survival, intimate relationships, and effective behaviors (Perls, 1959; Rogers, 1951, 1957).
2. *Holism:* People are made up of meaningful total patterns and wholes influenced by their environments (Mann, 2021).
3. *Field theory:* People interact in the here and now with their external environment, known as a situation (Mann, 2021). Sandtray scenes are part of a client's situation.
4. *Awareness, contact, and contact boundaries:* People have access to their immediate sense of what is and make meaning of their reciprocal contact with their environment (Mann, 2021; Perls, Hefferline, & Goodman, 1951/1994). Contact boundaries allow people to self-regulate amid supportive or toxic environments (Polster & Polster, 1973). Increased awareness is explained by the awareness-excitement-contact cycle (Zinker, 1977).
5. *Freedom and responsibility:* People are free to choose within context of their situation and are ultimately responsible for choices they make (Cain, 2002).

Client–Therapist Relationship

Humanistic sandtray therapists are facilitators of sandtray therapy and maintain that clients are the experts of their own worlds. In HST, the therapeutic relationship is regarded as a necessary but insufficient condition for client change to occur, and development of a deep therapeutic relationship must precede introduction of HST as a therapeutic approach to clients. In HST, the nature of the therapeutic relationship parallels Rogers' (1957) conceptualization captured in the core conditions of client change: psychological contact created and maintained by therapist and client; client arrives incongruent; therapist maintains congruence, genuineness, and realness; therapist experiences unconditional positive regard; therapist experiences and communicates empathy; and client experiences and accepts therapist's unconditional positive regard and empathy.

There are two gestalt concepts that further the client–therapist relationship in HST. Dialogue is a kind of contact that happens when therapist and client reach out to each other in an authentic manner to affect each other (Yontef, 1993). Inclusion is like empathy but is an experience in which the therapist maintains a deeper sense of the client's perspective while feeling a more intense existential separateness.

Theoretical Mechanisms of Action

The mechanisms of action in HST are based on the paradoxical theory of change: "*change occurs when one becomes what [one] is, not when [one] tries*

Copyright material from Ryan D. Foster (2025), *Humanistic Sandtray Therapy*, Routledge

to become what [one] is not" (Beisser, 1970, p. 77, italics theirs). Therapists do not directly create change in clients; rather, they work with clients to co-create a situation that brings a client to who, what, and how they are by opening a therapeutic environment that welcomes clients to decrease their defensiveness and increase self-awareness.

HST posits that learning and change is experiential. A specific kind of learning, increased awareness, exposes clients to options to respond to their own internal processes as well as external environments. In HST, awareness is always couched in the here and now. During therapy, therapists focus on "*what* clients are experiencing and *how* they experience it" (Armstrong et al., 2017, p. 221; italics theirs).

In HST, sandtray promotes experiential awareness and leads to change based on five elements:

1. *Sensory experiencing*: Kinesthetic awareness is activated during HST when clients touch and manipulate the sand and the miniatures, as well as during bodywork.
2. *Indirect expression and inclusivity*: Clients express their narratives and experiences by creating sandtray scenes, allowing them to communicate non-verbally.
3. *Catharsis*: Clients' deep or hidden emotions can be provoked by creating and processing their sandtray scenes.
4. *Metaphor*: Clients create their own metaphors, allowing them to observe their own experiences from a new point of view.
5. *Therapeutic depth*: HST "fosters deeper self-disclosure" (Armstrong, 2008, p. 12) due to its focus on metaphor, indirect expression, sensory experiencing, and cathartic experiencing.

Appropriate Populations for HST

HST is appropriate for clients who are preadolescents to adults, functional ages 10 and up. Sandtray does not rely solely on client verbalization for clients to benefit therapeutically. Developmentally, clients who are cognitively in concrete operations phase but who demonstrate beginning capacities for formal operations are appropriate. Sandtray has concrete and abstract elements, and metaphor can act as a storytelling mechanism for people who are transitioning to formal operations.

Empirical Evidence Supporting the Effectiveness of HST

Currently, HST has no research supporting its core technical elements. Generally, sandtray therapy is supported by cross-theoretical research (Homeyer & Sweeney, 2023). Four prior treatment outcome studies have

Copyright material from Ryan D. Foster (2025), *Humanistic Sandtray Therapy*, Routledge

provided initial support for the effectiveness of humanistically oriented sandtray approaches in school-aged preadolescents and adolescents. Flahive and Ray (2007) investigated the effect of group person-centered sandtray therapy on problematic behaviors, internalizing problems, and externalizing problems of preadolescents. They found a statistically significant difference and medium effect size between the experimental and control groups on measures of problematic behavior and internalizing and externaling behaviors, indicating a moderately effectual impact of group person-centered sandtray therapy. Nelson-Ray (2007) explored the impact of Lowenfeld's (2007) World Technique on academic achievement, school satisfaction, problematic behaviors, and school attendance rates of at-risk adolescents in group counseling. She found statistically significant differences between the treatment and control groups on a state mathematics achievement test and school satisfaction, and no differences with school attendance rates and problematic behaviors. Shen and Armstrong (2008) researched the impact of group HST on self-esteem of females in seventh grade. They found statistically significant and medium to large effect sizes on multiple subscales of a self-esteem measure, noting that group humanistic sandtray therapy can be beneficial for the self-esteem of preadolescent and young adolescent girls. Finally, Plotkin (2011) investigated the impact of individual child-centered sandtray play therapy on internalizing and externalizing problems of children aged 6 to 10 years old who were experiencing parental divorce. She found a significantly significant difference between the treatment and wait-list control groups on measures of internalizing and externalizing behaviors, indicating that sandtray had a positive impact on participants.

Specification of Defining Interventions

Elements and Interventions Shared with Other Sandtray Approaches

HST shares many practical elements with other approaches to sandtray therapy. Specifically, the types of sand trays and miniatures used mirror those that Homeyer and Sweeney (2023) described. In addition, therapists provide clients a prompt that guides an area of focus for the sandtray that clients create. Prompts can be general, such as, "Build your life as you perceive it in the tray," to specific, such as, "Create a scene that depicts how you experience your depression." Furthermore, basic counseling skills such as reflection of feelings, reflection of non-verbals, and therapeutic silence are important to effective HST practice.

Copyright material from Ryan D. Foster (2025), *Humanistic Sandtray Therapy*, Routledge

Elements and Interventions Unique to HST

There are elements of HST that are unique and set this system apart from other sandtray approaches. Humanistic sandtray therapists regularly incorporate gestalt-oriented experiments and skills facilitative of increased awareness:

1. *Descriptive/exploratory questions:* Asking open-ended questions that encourage client to describe or notice how they are responding emotionally.
2. *Accentuating the obvious:* Asking client to exaggerate a feeling or body movement or directing client to repeat a figural statement.
3. *Facilitating owning experiences through language:* Directing client to use I-language as replacement for second-person when describing self, present tense to replace past tense, or replace "can't" with choice-oriented language.
4. *Enactment:* Directing client to dramatize a statement, gesture, or element of the sandtray scene.
5. *Facilitating body awareness:* Directing client to identify emotions and/or experiences in their body.
6. *Metaphor work:* Staying in the metaphor of the sandtray scene.
7. *Identifying, naming, and acknowledging polarities:* Facilitating initial identification and naming of a polarity and verifies with client accuracy of polarity.
8. *Separating and exploring parts of polarities:* Assessing and identifying presence of opposing parts in the here and now.
9. *Responding to resistance:* Working with client resistance using the polarities response model.

Copyright material from Ryan D. Foster (2025), *Humanistic Sandtray Therapy*, Routledge

Phases of HST

There are five distinct phases of HST. Some take place in the same session, whereas others take place over the longer term depending on the course of therapy. The five phases are: pre-creation, creation, processing, post-creation, and clean-up. These phases are described in Table A.1.

Table A.1 Five phases of HST

Phase	Major Elements	Therapeutic Tasks
Pre-creation	Client makes initial contact with the sand tray and miniatures.	Familiarize client with sandtray by introducing them to the tray, miniatures, and how it might help them with their issue(s).
Creation	Client clarifies awareness of figure and therapeutic need. Client creates sandtray scene.	Invite client into a short centering exercise to ground client. Provide a sandtray prompt.
Processing	Client experiences increased awareness via interventions focused on here and now.	Enter intervention phase of HST.
Post-creation	This phase often carries on into subsequent therapy sessions as client continues to reflect on new awareness gained.	Exit and reflect on the sandtray experience.
Clean-up	Client experientially withdraws from immediate sandtray experience.	Take a picture of the tray. Terminate session. Therapist dismantles tray after client leaves.

Copyright material from Ryan D. Foster (2025), *Humanistic Sandtray Therapy*, Routledge

General Format of HST

Primarily, HST is delivered individually. However, HST can be integrated as an adjunct to ongoing couples, family, and group therapy (open- or closed-ended). Because therapists use HST as indicated by client need, it can be used one time, several times over the course of therapy, or as the main therapeutic intervention.

Length of HST sessions varies depending on the client's development and the therapist's clinical setting. Pre-adolescents and young adolescents (<15 years old) can create and process a sandtray scene in as little as 30 minutes. Older adolescents (15 and up) and adults typically require a 50-minute session at minimum, and adults can often benefit from 90-minute sessions. Couples sandtray sessions are 90-minutes at minimum. Family sessions are two to three hours, depending on the number of family members.

Copyright material from Ryan D. Foster (2025), *Humanistic Sandtray Therapy*, Routledge

Therapist Selection, Training, and Supervision

Therapist Selection and Training

Therapists who wish to become effective humanistic sandtray therapists embody the following ideal personal characteristics and experiences:

1. They remain open to their own internal experiencing of emotions and associated thoughts. They seek opportunities for self-awareness and growth.
2. They have attended their own psychotherapy to resolve unfinished business.
3. They are open to vulnerability and can access compassion and empathy with relative ease.
4. They are attuned to their own microawareness (awareness of awareness).

Therapists who aim to practice HST must receive formal training from an HST-certified trainer through the Humanistic Sandtray Therapy Institute. This training consists of Level I and Level II/Advanced training modules. Each module consists of 15 continuing education credit hours (CEs) of training, for a total of 30 CEs. Table A.2 shows the core elements of each training level.

Table A.2 Core elements of Level I and Level II training

Level I	Level II
• Learn the basics of sandtray including conducting a session, determining clients appropriate for the modality, understanding of rationale for sandtray, and practical matters such as acquisition of miniatures. • Become more proficient at understanding and practicing humanistic sandtray processing through live demonstrations, experiential activities, and group discussion. • Improve ability to respond to non-verbal, here-and-now expressions of emotion, work effectively in the here and now, see and respond to polarities, and facilitate awareness and depth of experiencing.	• Continue to develop ability to respond to non-verbal expressions of emotion in sandtray, work effectively in the here and now, see and respond to polarities, and facilitate awareness and depth of experiencing. • Enhance self-awareness, experience emotion in the moment, and gain insight into personal issues that may hinder client growth if not addressed. • Learn how to gently guide sandtray clients to a deeper level of experiencing.

Copyright material from Ryan D. Foster (2025), *Humanistic Sandtray Therapy*, Routledge

Table A.2 (Continued)

Level I	Level II
• Enhance self-awareness, experience emotion in the moment, and gain insight into personal issues that may hinder client growth if not addressed. • Receive supervision and feedback during group sandtray experiences and observations.	• Demonstrate the ability to utilize a descriptive mode of responding that helps clients to explore emotions and avoid analysis and explanations of inner experiencing. • Learn to recognize, identify, separate, and work effectively with both sides of polarities. • Learn the humanistic approach to working with resistance, including the following: Recognizing physical blocks and responding in ways that help the client feel safer; gently guiding clients through a process of awareness of their defenses in the here and now; and helping clients to utilize ways of their defenses increasing tension before relaxing such as accentuating the obvious.

Copyright material from Ryan D. Foster (2025), *Humanistic Sandtray Therapy*, Routledge

HST Supervision

It is highly recommended that therapists seek credentials as a Certified Humanistic Sandtray Therapy (CHST), for which they undergo post-training HST supervision. The minimum number of supervision hours required for the CHST credential is ten. HST supervisees are required to create a minimum of five sandtrays of their own. Also, supervisees are required to videorecord a minimum of five HST sessions with clients and submit them for observation and evaluation by their HST supervisor.

Evaluating Adherence and Competence

There are training tools available for adherents of HST. Two books are primary sources for learning the theory and therapeutic conditions of this method (Armstrong, 2008; Foster, 2025). In addition, the Humanistic Sandtray Therapy Institute's website (https://humanisticsandtray.com/videos) makes available several videos that demonstrate use of HST with various client populations and formats.

In clinical settings, HST supervisors evaluate therapist adherence and competence using the Humanistic Sandtray Therapy Session Evaluation (HST-SE). Supervisors can use this form to evaluate videorecorded HST sessions when they observe them either during or outside of supervision sessions. The HST-SE assesses 14 core skills and strategies used in HST on a Likert-type scale of 1 to 5. Lower numbers indicate inappropriate levels of HST skills, and higher numbers indicate appropriate levels of HST skills. Each skill is assigned a rating.

Copyright material from Ryan D. Foster (2025), *Humanistic Sandtray Therapy*, Routledge

Humanistic Sandtray Therapy Session Evaluation (HST-SE)

Supervisor: _____   Therapist: _____   Client Age: _____

1	2	3	4	5
Skills used inappropriately according to HST protocol		Skill used moderately appropriately according to HST protocol		Skill used appropriately according to HST protocol

HST Skill						Comments
Provided a sandtray prompt responsive to client needs	1	2	3	4	5	
Reflecting feelings (in the present tense)	1	2	3	4	5	
Reflecting non-verbal expressions of emotion (client gestures, facial expressions, body position)	1	2	3	4	5	
Immediacy/here and now responses (responds to client's in the moment content and process)	1	2	3	4	5	
Therapeutic silence (paired with empathic facial expression to encourage client to stay with their present emotion)	1	2	3	4	5	
Asking descriptive/exploratory questions (open-ended questions that encourage client to describe or notice how they are responding emotionally)	1	2	3	4	5	
Accentuating the obvious (asks client to exaggerate a feeling or body movement, or directs client to repeat a figural statement)	1	2	3	4	5	
Facilitating owning experiences through language (directs client to: use I-language as replacement for second person when describing self, use present tense to replace past tense, or replace "can't" with choice-oriented language)	1	2	3	4	5	

Copyright material from Ryan D. Foster (2025), *Humanistic Sandtray Therapy*, Routledge

HST Skill						Comments
Enactment (directs client to dramatize a statement, gesture, or element of the sandtray scene)	1	2	3	4	5	
Facilitating body awareness (directs client to identify emotions and/or experiences in their body)	1	2	3	4	5	
Metaphor work (facilitates staying in the metaphor of the sandtray scene)	1	2	3	4	5	
Responding to polarities: Identifying, naming, and acknowledging (facilitates initial identification and naming of the polarity and verifies with client accuracy of polarity)	1	2	3	4	5	
Responding to polarities: Separating and exploring parts (assesses and identifies presence of opposing parts in the here and now)	1	2	3	4	5	
Responding to resistance (works with client resistance using polarities response model)	1	2	3	4	5	

In research settings, HST researchers use the Humanistic Sandtray Therapy Treatment Fidelity Measure (HST-TFM) to ensure treatment fidelity. It is used to rate core requisite HST skills demonstrated on videorecorded HST sessions on a scale of 1—not present, 2—minimally present, and 3—optimally present. This instrument is early in its development and requires further validation to ensure it is capturing fidelity appropriately.

Copyright material from Ryan D. Foster (2025), *Humanistic Sandtray Therapy*, Routledge

Humanistic Sandtray Therapy Treatment Fidelity Measure (HST-TFM)

Rater: _____ Therapist ID: _____ Client ID: _____

Session ID: _____ Start Time: _____ End Time: _____

Rating Scale: 1—Not present 2—Minimally present 3—Optimally present

Therapist's Responses	Skill Demonstration Level			
Session ID: _____ Start Time: ____ End Time: ___				
Therapist's Responses	Skill Demonstration Level			Notes
Reflecting Feelings Therapist reflects client emotions using present tense.	1	2	3	
Reflecting Non-verbal Expressions of Emotion Therapist reflects client gestures, facial expressions, body position.	1	2	3	
Immediacy/Here-and-Now Responses Therapist responds to client's in the moment content and process.	1	2	3	
Therapeutic Silence Therapist uses therapeutic silence paired with empathic facial expression to encourage client to stay with their present emotion(s).	1	2	3	
Asking Descriptive/ Exploratory Questions Therapist asks open-ended questions that encourage client to describe or notice how they are responding emotionally.	1	2	3	
Accentuating the Obvious Therapist asks client to exaggerate a feeling or body movement or directs client to repeat a figural statement.	1	2	3	

Copyright material from Ryan D. Foster (2025), *Humanistic Sandtray Therapy*, Routledge

Therapist's Responses	Skill Demonstration Level			Notes
Facilitating Owning Experiences through Language Therapist directs client to use I-language as replacement for second person when describing self, use present tense to replace past tense, or replace "can't" with choice-oriented language (e.g., won't, unwilling to, choose to).	1	2	3	
Enactment Therapist directs client to dramatize a statement, gesture, or element of the sandtray scene.	1	2	3	
Facilitating Body Awareness Therapist directs client to identify emotions and/or experiences in their body.	1	2	3	
Metaphor Work Therapist facilitates staying in the metaphor of the sandtray scene: Level 1—asks client to describe scene. Level 2—offers observations about the scene. Level 3—invites client into the metaphor/scene. Level 4—personalizes metaphor and connects to client's clinical themes/issues.	1	2	3	
Responding to Polarities: Identifying, Naming, and Acknowledging Therapist facilitates initial identification and naming of the polarity and verifies with client accuracy of polarity.	1	2	3	
Responding to Polarities: Separating and Exploring Parts Therapist identifies presence of opposing parts in the here and now.	1	2	3	

Copyright material from Ryan D. Foster (2025), *Humanistic Sandtray Therapy*, Routledge

Therapist's Responses	Skill Demonstration Level			Notes
Non-HST Response Response that does not fit clearly into the categories above.	1	2	3	
Unintelligible Responses Responses that the rater cannot hear well or cannot understand.	1	2	3	

Copyright material from Ryan D. Foster (2025), *Humanistic Sandtray Therapy*, Routledge

References

Armstrong, S. A. (2008). *Sandtray therapy: A humanistic approach*. Ludic Press.

Armstrong, S. A., Foster, R. D., Brown, T., & Davis, J. (2017). Humanistic sandtray therapy with children and adults. In E. S. Leggett & J. N. Boswell (Eds.), *Directive play therapy: Theories and techniques* (pp. 217–253). Springer.

Beisser, A. (1970). The paradoxical theory of change. In J. Fagan & I. L. Shepherd (Eds.), *Gestalt therapy now: Theories, techniques, applications* (pp. 77–80). Science and Behavior Books.

Cain, D. J. (2002). Defining characteristics, history, and evolution of humanistic psychotherapies. In D. J. Cain & J. Seeman (Eds.), *Humanistic psychotherapies: Handbook of research and practice* (pp. 3–54). American Psychological Association.

Flahive, M. H. W., & Ray, D. (2007). Effect of group sandtray therapy with preadolescents. *The Journal for Specialists in Group Work, 32*(4), 362–382. https://doi.org/10.1080/01933920701476706

Foster, R. D. (2025). *Humanistic sandtray therapy: The definitive guide to philosophy, therapeutic conditions, and the real relationship*. Routledge.

Herlihy, B. (1985). Person-centered gestalt therapy: A synthesis. *Journal of Humanistic Education and Development, 24*(1), 16–24. https://doi.org/10.1002/j.2164-4683.1985.tb00274.x

Homeyer, L. E., & Sweeney, D. S. (2023). *Sandtray therapy: A practical manual* (4th ed.). Routledge. https://doi.org/10.4324/9781003221418

Lowenfeld, M. (2007). *Understanding children's sandplay: Lowenfeld's World Technique*. Sussex Academic Press.

Mann, D. (2021). *Gestalt therapy: 100 key points and techniques* (2nd ed.). Routledge. https://doi.org/10.4324/9781315158495

Nelson-Ray, P. (2007). *Using sand tray with at-risk students to impact school success* [Unpublished doctoral dissertation]. Texas Tech University.

Perls, F. S. (1959). *Gestalt therapy verbatim*. Real People Press.

Perls, F., Hefferline, R., & Goodman, P. (1951/1994). *Gestalt therapy: Excitement and growth in the human personality*. The Gestalt Journal Press.

Plotkin, L. (2011). Children's adjustment following parental divorce: How effective is sandtray therapy? [Unpublished doctoral dissertation]. Capella University.

Polster, E., & Polster, M. (1973). *Gestalt therapy integrated: Contours of theory & practice*. Brunner/Mazel.

Rogers, C. R. (1951). *Client-centered therapy: Its current practice, implications and theory*. Houghton-Mifflin.

Rogers, C. R. (1957). The necessary and sufficient conditions of therapeutic personality change. *Journal of Consulting Psychology, 21*(2), 95–103. https://psycnet.apa.org/doi/10.1037/h0045357

Shen, Y. P., & Armstrong, S. A. (2008). Impact of group sandtray therapy on the self-esteem of young adolescent girls. *The Journal for Specialists in Group Work, 33*(2), 118–137. https://doi.org/10.1080/ 01933920801977397

Yontef, G. (1993). *Awareness, dialogue & process*. The Gestalt Press.

Zinker, J. (1977). *Creative process in Gestalt therapy*. Brunner/Mazel.

Index

For Product Safety Concerns and Information please contact our EU representative GPSR@taylorandfrancis.com Taylor & Francis Verlag GmbH, Kaufingerstraße 24, 80331 München, Germany